YES|NO

YES|NO

USING THE
ARM-LENGTH TEST
FOR INSTANT ANSWERS
AND WELLBEING

UWE ALBRECHT MD

HAY HOUSE

Australia • Canada • Hong Kong • India
South Africa • United Kingdom • United States

First published and distributed in the United Kingdom by:
Hay House UK Ltd, 292B Kensal Rd, London W10 5BE.
Tel.: (44) 20 8962 1230; Fax: (44) 20 8962 1239.
www.hayhouse.co.uk

Published and distributed in the United States of America by:
Hay House, Inc., PO Box 5100, Carlsbad, CA 92018-5100.
Tel.: (1) 760 431 7695 or (800) 654 5126;
Fax: (1) 760 431 6948 or (800) 650 5115.
www.hayhouse.com

Published and distributed in Australia by:
Hay House Australia Ltd, 18/36 Ralph St, Alexandria NSW 2015.
Tel.: (61) 2 9669 4299; Fax: (61) 2 9669 4144.
www.hayhouse.com.au

Published and distributed in the Republic of South Africa by:
Hay House SA (Pty), Ltd, PO Box 990, Witkoppen 2068.
Tel./Fax: (27) 11 467 8904. www.hayhouse.co.za

Published and distributed in India by:
Hay House Publishers India, Muskaan Complex, Plot No.3, B-2,
Vasant Kunj, New Delhi – 110 070. Tel.: (91) 11 4176 1620; Fax: (91) 11 4176 1630.
www.hayhouse.co.in

Distributed in Canada by:
Raincoast, 9050 Shaughnessy St, Vancouver, BC V6P 6E5.
Tel.: (1) 604 323 7100; Fax: (1) 604 323 2600

Text © Uwe Albrecht, 2012

The information given in this book should not be treated as a substitute for professional
medical advice; always consult a medical practitioner. Any use of information in this book is at
the reader's discretion and risk. Neither the author nor the publisher can be held responsible
for any loss, claim or damage arising out of the use, or misuse, of the suggestions made or the
failure to take medical advice, or for any material on third party websites.

Translated by Irina Pálffy-Daun-Seiler with assistance from Valerie Linares.

A catalogue record for this book is available from the British Library

ISBN: 978-1-84850-975-7

Interior images: 34, 35, 40b, 41b, 42b, 43b, 44c © istockphoto; all other photography and
illustration: Anna Badowska, Silke Kröger, Katharina Kosak, Eric Frank and Leanne Sui Anastasi

Thank you, Raphael van Assche,
for your spirit of discovery
and your gift of this test.

CONTENTS

Chapter 1: The Arm-Length Test

Chapter 2: Key Test Questions

Chapter 3: Using the Arm-Length Test Throughout the Day

Chapter 4: The Arm-Length Test in All Life Situations

The Arm-Length Test for Health

The Arm-Length Test for Happiness and Wellbeing

CONTENTS

If I were a tree, I would drink the water around me. I would move as the wind touched me, nourish myself from the shining sun, and live with the wounds of the knives that carved hearts into my bark.

If I were water, I would let myself float. I would join with other water, turn into steam if I sweated, and into ice if I froze.

If I were a bird, I would be able to fly, to walk and sometimes dive. I would be free and go anywhere I wanted to.

But I'm a human being.

And as long as I'm human, I always have a choice whether or not to do something, when to do it and how to do it. At any moment, I may find myself at a crossroads and have to make a decision. Sometimes I make good decisions, and sometimes I don't. At times, my intuition guides me, and at other times I let outside voices influence me. Everything else is coincidence.

There are main roads if I want to take a safe route; there are green lanes if I want to breathe the fresh air of freedom; and there are meadows if I want to pick flowers.

And then there is our inner wisdom, which can guide us. We encounter it as our gut feeling, as a hunch, as a vision, and as the arm-length test, which expresses itself in a change in the length of our arms when we say 'yes' or 'no'.

Yes or No! The ONE thing life is NOT is 'maybe'!

Chapter 1

THE ARM-LENGTH TEST

YES OR NO, BUT NEVER MAYBE

You are either pregnant or you aren't – you can't be 'maybe' pregnant. In a restaurant, you have to make a choice and order. At a traffic intersection, you can't move forward unless you pick a direction.

This is our lot as human beings. In each situation, we have to make a decision:

- What should I wear today?

- What should I have for breakfast?

- Do I need to take any vitamins today?

- Is there a traffic jam today? Which is the fastest route to work?

- What should I do first today at work?

- What should I buy at the supermarket, and what can I tolerate?

3

- How should I decorate my home?

- Should I put fresh flowers in this room?

- Should I go and see a doctor for my back pain?

- What should I do when I have a cold?

- Should I still go to the movies today?

Questions, questions, questions, and constant decisions – this is our lot as human beings.

The price for our freedom is self-responsibility.

THE MIND OR THE SUBCONSCIOUS – WHO DECIDES?

You may think the mind is important. You may believe that with our minds we can achieve almost anything. I also used to think this way.

Until the moment when I started to test all the patients at my doctor's practice using the arm-length test.

I asked all of them to imagine the same thing – being healthy.

And then I asked them to imagine the opposite – remaining ill.

I was shocked by the result, and suddenly I saw the world in a new light.

People had driven for hours to come and see me for a treatment. They had already tried numerous therapies and they were willing to pay for them out of their own pockets. And all of these people declared they had just one wish: finally to be healthy again.

Yet they all, without exception, revealed stress through the arm-length test when they imagined being healthy. Their bodies screamed 'NO!', but then they all revealed a 'YES' as they imagined themselves remaining ill.

I saw the same results when working with couples hoping to conceive. They all showed maximum stress when asked to imagine being pregnant. How was this supposed to work if they couldn't even imagine it?

Statements such as, 'We've tried everything for the past ten years' weren't of any help here either.

Usually, couples hoping to conceive who come to see me for a treatment are able to conceive about two weeks later. Naturally, this only works if both partners can imagine the pregnancy on a subconscious level – i.e. if the arm-length test shows a 'yes' to the pregnancy for both partners.

5

We encounter the same problem of inner sabotage in unhappy, unsuccessful people, or in involuntarily single people. It's always the same: the mind says 'yes' and the subconscious says 'no'.

Consequently, I started to test the actual share of the conscious mind, compared to the subconscious, in decision-making in our lives.

Consistently, 90 per cent of all those tested showed the following results: 1 to 5 per cent for the conscious mind, and 95 to 99 per cent for the subconscious.

There were only a few exceptions, and all of them were very special people with a high level of consciousness reflected in their shining eyes and in their whole aura.

This made it clear to me that if we want to change something, we have to communicate and work with our subconscious.

THE BODY RESPONDS

Our bodies can talk. And they don't lie. Goosebumps, cold sweats, sexual arousal, the heart beating fast with excitement, yawning and sneezing to cleanse yourself of energies, inner vibrations caused by fear – all these responses are ways in which the body communicates to us.

Yet it can do a lot more than that. If we say, 'I can't resist you!', it's not only our resistance to a temptation that's weakened, our muscles also become weak.

We are made up of many rhythms – the heart rhythm, the breathing rhythm – and there are many more, although they are not listed in conventional medical books. And they change as well. There is our cranial breath, and that of our spine – the craniosacral rhythm. Our liver also has its own rhythm, and the same applies to our kidneys. Each organ has its own rhythm, its own vibration. And none of them remain constant. As we experience stress or balance, our breath and heartbeat get faster or slower. Our cranial breath changes, too, as well as the rhythm of each organ in our body.

We are like an instrument that sounds harmonious and beautiful if it's well tuned. Yet, when out of tune or out of balance, it sounds simply awful.

In mathematical terms, when we are in balance, in harmony, our vibration is sinusoidal.

When we feel stressed and are in a state of disharmony, it goes up and down, like a chaotically jagged curve seen on the stockmarket charts.

Then, in addition to harmony and disharmony, there is a third state: rigidity.

7

Here, although we are not officially dead, neither are we really alive anymore. We function merely in survival mode.

Do you think that disharmony or rigidity are rare? Not at all!

Most people living on this planet are in a state of disharmony, or to be precise, 59 per cent of them. And how many are half-dead, or to put it nicely, in survival mode? 26 per cent of all people are caught in this state of rigidity.

This leaves only 15 per cent of all people on this planet who manage to live in harmony.

These people are inwardly beautiful and therefore, for the most part, outwardly beautiful. They sound beautiful, they are able to feel well, be happy and enjoy good health on all levels: physically, mentally, emotionally and energetically.

Is that really what the Creator had in mind?

Hardly. With 85 per cent of people being unhappy, what a waste...

Go and take a conscious look at people on the street. How many of them look like they are in balance?

THE SIXTH SENSE: INTUITION

A good friend once said to me, 'I think I lost my sixth sense brooding about things.' The sixth sense is our ability to perceive something without grasping it consciously using our senses of sight, hearing, smell, taste and touch. The sixth sense is rich in impressions and ways of expression; it includes feeling and sensing, knowing something inside, having a hunch about something, and perceiving the feelings and thoughts of others, as well as clairvoyance, clairsentience and telepathy.

It's our intuition, a sense that's often considered already extinct, burned at the stakes of the Inquisition.

Yet, just as love cannot be exterminated, the sixth sense has remained in every human being. It has merely been internally banished – barred behind all the blockages of our lives.

In the course of my workshops, I have shown many people the arm-length test. So far, everybody has been able to learn it, even those men who had entrenched themselves behind an inner armour of steel, convinced they couldn't feel anything.

I rediscovered my own intuition when I was 32 years old by using the arm-length test. I was able to help my older children to rediscover it, and with my younger children I was able to prevent it from fading away. As a result, my children are able to see energy fields, to know what's good for them and what isn't, and to sense the intentions of other people.

Intuition can influence systems and entire countries – it can have an effect on policy-making per se. It enables us to differentiate truth from lies and to determine our lives for ourselves.

The body has no organ like the eyes, ears, tongue or skin for the sixth sense. In fact, the entire body serves as the organ sensing our intuition, our inner wisdom.

We feel it in our guts, the hair on our skin stands up, our breath falters... we receive many signs.

But what these signs have in common is that they are very individual and not always readily perceivable. They are often well hidden behind the masks that we feel we need in order to exist in this world. This means that we have to relearn to open up our bodily senses and to listen to these very fine perceptions during the course of our lives. For that, we need silence, silence within us, as these signs are often very faint.

There is also the reaction of our muscular system. It always occurs and it works in the same way in every human being. And It's visible in all life situations: a change in the length of our arms.

KINESIOLOGY, PENDULUMS AND MORE

There are several ways to render our intuition visible and test it: using instruments or devices, muscle reflexes and energy fields. Below you will find a brief overview of the different methods:

The Pendulum

Using a pendulum works because the direction in which the energy field of the palm rotates changes with a 'yes' or a 'no' statement. Depending on the state of the energy field, the movements may be circular or linear.

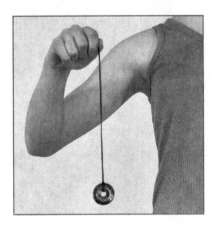

The pendulum

Pendulums, along with dowsing rods and biotensors, are fine antennas used to make changes in the visible energy field. By themselves – without the user's palm – they are nothing more than metal, wood, string or stones.

Dowsing Rods

Whether dowsing rods are made of wood or metal, they merely react to the energy field of the palm as well; they may cross over one another, or point in opposite directions, or they may dip or move upward.

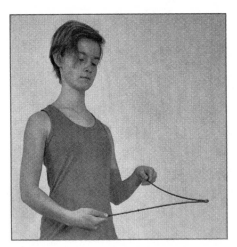

Dowsing rods: Y-rod

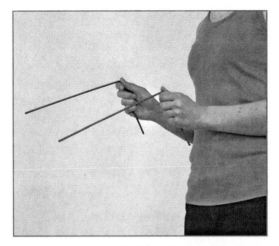

Dowsing rods: L-rod in balance

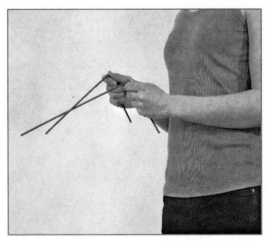

Dowsing rods: L-rod revealing stress

The Biotensor

Biotensors are very sensitive testing instruments. In some products, sensitivity is tangibly amplified by using coiled wire inside the handle. The biotensor reacts to changes in the energy field of the user's palm. Depending on the user's energy, they may swing horizontally or vertically, or move in a circular fashion.

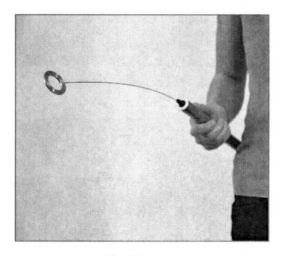

The Biotensor

The Lecher Antenna

The Lecher antenna is a hollow antenna rod that was developed by the Austrian physicist Ernst Lecher. Using a mobile cursor, the resonating space can be adjusted, thereby setting the antenna to specific frequencies. It's like tuning a radio. This antenna is also used manually.

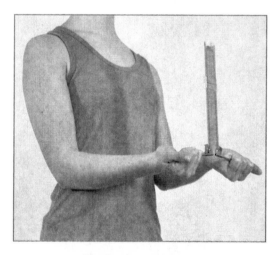

The Lecher antenna

The Muscle Test

The kinesiological muscle test is widely known and used. With a negative statement, a strong muscle becomes weak. Even the strongest man on Earth cannot hold up his arm against pressure while thinking of something negative.

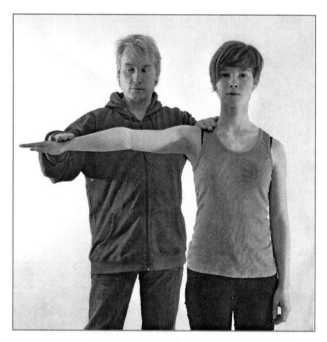

Strong muscle

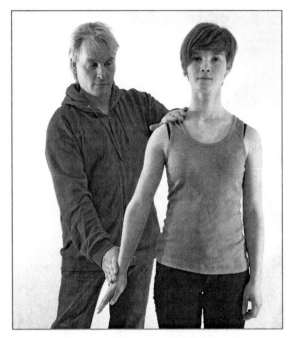

Weak muscle

The problem with this muscle test is that you cannot do it by yourself. There always has to be a second person who applies counterpressure.

The O-Ring Test

In the o-ring test, the thumb and index finger on both hands form an o-ring. These o-rings are linked, as in a chain. Trying to pry open the chain links while holding the o-rings together with maximum strength works only with a weakening 'no' statement.

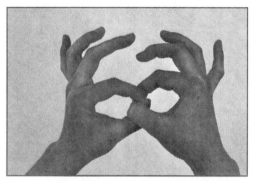

O-ring test: strong

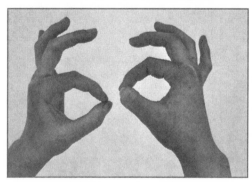

O-ring test: weak

The Pulse Test

Pulse testing is mainly applied by ear acupuncturists. They feel the pulse wave at the wrist, which changes with a 'no' statement. The autonomic nervous system changes the vessel width, thereby affecting pulse wave propagation; the pulse wave is being deformed, the interval between the two peaks may be longer, or it may have two peaks when you feel it with your fingers.

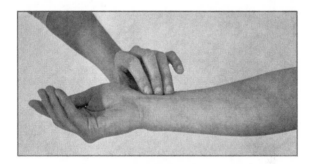

Pulse test

The Standing or Sway Test

The standing or sway test is very easy. You stand up, close your eyes, and feel your stance. With a positive statement, your weight will move slightly forward – you will sway forward. With a negative statement, your weight will move backward – you will sway backward. You are like a large pendulum.

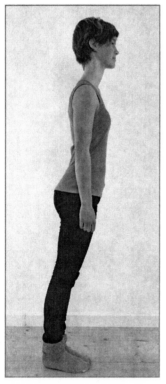 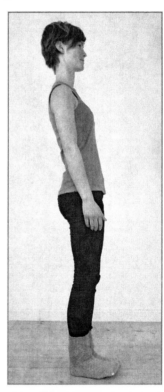

Standing or sway test: 'yes'   *Standing or sway test: 'no'*

Technical Systems

There are also technical systems that measure energetic changes in the body.

The oldest and most widely known is electro-acupuncture, which measures changes in resistance at acupuncture points as a result of stress.

More modern systems often originate from space or military research. They test frequencies sent through the body, as well as the body's responses. You can imagine this as like ultrasound. In this way, it's possible to measure the frequencies of organs and compare them to databases to determine which pattern they correspond to. These are the most expensive tests.

WHAT IS THE ARM-LENGTH TEST?

The arm-length test is the most sensitive and diverse testing system:

- It doesn't cost a thing.

- Anyone can apply it by him- or herself.

- It's with us wherever we go.

- Children can use it too!

- We no longer delegate testing to a tool, instead, we trust our bodies.

- The arm-length test can do a lot more than just express a 'yes' or a 'no'.

- It reveals how big the stress is – a small 'no', a medium 'no' or a big 'no'.

- It reveals whether we are out of balance in general.

- It indicates whether we are free or caught in a state of rigidity.

- It shows even when we are panicking, or allergic to something.

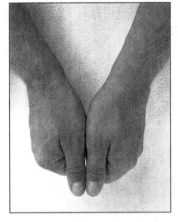

Arm-length test: 'yes', or balance

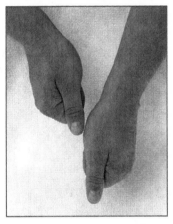

Arm-length test: 'no', or stress

Handcrafted, tried and tested, can't be replaced by a pendulum or a computer system.

HOW DOES THE ARM-LENGTH TEST WORK?

This is not some esoteric fad. It's a neurological reflex, with the muscles relaxing on one side of the body while they are contracting on the other. This is why the arms differ in length.

It's a response of our muscular system to stress. Here, the brain controls our muscles via a neuropeptide, the substance P, at the speed of 1,500 metres (about a mile) per second, in ways that make strong muscles suddenly become weak.

As a physician, I test everything by checking the length of the arms. In what state are the organs? How high is the level of life energy? Which childhood trauma has not been resolved yet? Which medication helps? Does the patient have an allergic reaction to any dental material? To start with, does the patient really want to be healthy again?

The test connects mind and heart. In this way, the heart can communicate truths to the sceptical mind that aren't otherwise graspable on a logical level.

HOW THE ARM-LENGTH TEST FOUND ME

Even if I still believed in coincidences, there were too many of their kind for me not to recognize serendipity as the driving force.

I'm a physician, and in addition to conventional medicine, I'd studied many alternative healing methods. At the time, I found myself in front of patients asking myself which would be the most effective therapy to help them.

So I started to test the different therapies, first using a pendulum, then a biotensor and then the Lecher antenna.

Freely based on the motto 'Once the reputation's shot, you get away with quite a lot!' I started to use the biotensor directly in my treatments. This was less unusual to my patients than it was to me.

I guess I was a bit slow, as it took a third broken biotensor metal tip for me to realize that I no longer needed this instrument. In fact, I'd used it to project the patient's response onto it. The time of 'the pendulum said...' was over. Using the arms was sufficient.

Back to handcraft.

Numerous 'coincidences' led me to a teacher of physioenergetics. He taught the arm-length test that the Belgian osteopath Raphael van Assche had discovered.

Many years ago, Raphael van Assche examined a woman's muscle chains. She was lying on her back and he pulled her arms up above her head. They were equally long. Then the woman started to talk about her husband, and about their enormous problems. Suddenly, her arms differed in length without any effort on her part. This was the beginning. And nowadays thousands of therapists use this test in their work.

I started to use the arm-length test immediately in my practice, and I also taught it to my patients so they would be able to help themselves if they needed to.

This was in 1996. It was the beginning of a journey of discovery and of a great love.

Since then, I've developed *Innerwise®: The Complete Healing System*, which comprises a book, cards and an amulet. Together with a team of trained mentors, I've taught the arm-length test to thousands of people and they have also learned how to treat themselves with Innerwise, a system which enables anyone to balance him- or herself. *Innerwise®: The Complete Healing System* is published by Hay House.

WHO RESPONDS TO THE ARM-LENGTH TEST?

At first, we could think it's the conscious mind.

But, contrary to this is the fact that:

1. The test works perfectly on coma patients. No one would seriously argue that their responses come from the conscious mind. It's for good reason that the coma state is referred to as 'unconscious'.

2. The test also works with cats and dogs, and some therapists have even used it with horses.

3. The test works with people and animals even if the test question is just written on a piece of paper and placed on the body of the person or animal, or when an independent tester merely *thinks* of the question.

4. It works when the testee is sleeping.

5. Even babies can be tested.

6. Often, the response is the exact opposite of what the person is thinking.

All this supports my point that the response doesn't come from the conscious mind.

If we don't assume right away that God is talking to us through our arms, the subconscious – our dialogue partner – remains the only source of the response. Another phenomenon occurs when trained testers receive the same response from a testee on a particular topic, without knowing each other's test results.

This applies not only to questions directed to people, but also to questions about situations and projects.

This raises the question as to whether the subconscious of each human being exists in isolation, or whether it's a common field where the subconscious of all people, or at least parts of it, meet and intermix.

I can't give a definite answer on who we talk to when using the arm-length test; the only thing I can say for sure is that it's not the conscious mind.

LEARNING HOW TO USE THE ARM-LENGTH TEST

The following step-by-step exercises will help you learn how to use the arm-length test and become confident in its use.

Step 1: Spherical Vision

You need a new type of vision in order to obtain reliable test results.

You have to learn to look at something from the outside. This also means seeing yourself from the outside if what you test is about you.

For how long did humanity believe that the Earth was flat and lay at the centre of the universe, and that the sun orbited the Earth? This happens when you look at something only from your own perspective, rather than independently from the outside.

You'll want to avoid this happening to you during testing – with the result that you test nonsense or half-truths – so the first thing you need to learn is a new way of seeing. This is called spherical vision.

It's very difficult to look at yourself from the outside, totally detached, as if you were not at all concerned about your fate.

Usually, we look at a topic or issue only from our perspective; this means that we only see a small part of the truth. And everyone sees something different.

If you apply this way of looking at someone or something, the response of the arm-length test is only 80 per cent correct, and thus useless.

To apply spherical vision, you can imagine standing in the middle of a large sphere. The sphere's shell is made up of eyes that you can observe yourself with.

Or, you can imagine that you are the Earth, and that you look at yourself from all directions, as if all the stars had eyes.

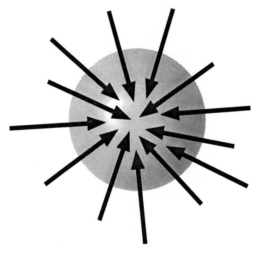

Spherical vision

Applying spherical vision isn't easy. For some people, it's the most difficult part of the arm-length test, because the tester should always apply this vision when testing.

And now you are ready to start practising:

1. Look at a bouquet of flowers. Look at one point only – a leaf, a stain or a blossom – and focus just on this one point.

2. Now change your perspective. Imagine you can see the bouquet of flowers from all directions: from the front, from behind, from above and below, and all of this at the same time. This is possible once you no longer look directly at one point, but instead focus on the space around the bouquet of flowers. As if you wanted to see its energy field.

3. Now switch back and forth a few times between these two perspectives and the way you see.

Only if you learn to see in this way can you really trust the arm-length test.

This means that you no longer see and judge from your own limited perspective and compare, but instead, seeing is independent from your own personal will.

Step 2: Sensing Colours

1. Imagine wearing clothes in different colours: purple, blue, orange, black, light green, red, yellow and white.

2. Sense the effect of the colours on you, and how they make you feel. Take a few minutes to do this.

3. Which colour makes you feel good?

4. What do the different colours change in you? What reaction do they trigger in you?

5. Now try this exercise with your eyes closed.

Step 3: Sensing 'Yes' and 'No'

Help! My body is talking to me!

1. No matter where you are at a given moment, stand in a relaxed way, tune in to yourself and feel:
    – your stance
    – your breath
    – your heart's rhythm
    – your aura
    – your energy field
    – your muscle tension
    – your body's rhythms

2. Now think of a beautiful situation that you've experienced in your life and sense how your body feels.

3. Then think of a bad, or even horrible, situation in your life and tune in again. You will perceive many differences within you.

4. Then say 'yes' out loud and tune in to yourself again.

5. Now say 'no' out loud and tune in once more. Does something change within you when you say 'no'?

6. Repeat this exercise a few more times, switching between 'yes' and 'no' until you're sure that you trust what you feel and that what you feel is real and you are not making it up.

You can also do this exercise in a seated position, although I recommend you repeat the exercise again later standing up, as some things can only be perceived in this position.

Step 4: I'm a Scale

1. Imagine you are a scale. Is the scale in balance, or out of balance?

2. If the scale is out of balance, imagine different colours again. Which colour restores the balance?

3. When you have identified the right colour, put on clothes in this colour, or just imagine doing this. It can also just be a scarf, a sock or a piece of coloured paper that you put in your pocket. If you can't balance your scale with any colour, take the colour that works best and imagine different scents. Both scents and colours together will rebalance your scale.

4. Or, you draw one to three healing cards from the *Innerwise®: The Complete Healing System* trusting your intuition. Then, you meditate with them. Trust yourself – you will always pick the right cards.

5. Continue only once you have restored your scale's balance.

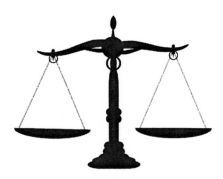

Scale in balance

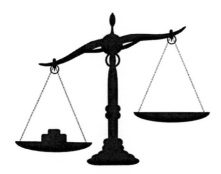

Scale slightly out of balance

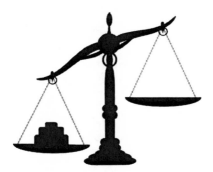

Scale severely out of balance

Congratulations! You have just treated yourself!

If your scale is in balance now, imagine adding a little weight on one side and observe how the scale moves. Then add a slightly heavier weight, followed by a really heavy one.

It's also possible that your scale is always in the same position, no matter how heavy the stone is that you add in your imagination. Then you are caught in a state of rigidity: you are blocked. Just as I described for the scale that was out of balance, you can also treat yourself in this situation. Using colours, scents or herbal teas will get you out of this state of rigidity.

In essence, testing is really simple:

- If we are in balance, our scale is in balance.

- If we are stressed, our scale is out of balance. It's like a scale with a weight on one side.

- If we are in a state of rigidity the scale doesn't move, regardless of whether it was in balance or out of balance when it entered that state. You are in a state of shock, frozen, caught in a trauma. The joy of life is lost, and life becomes a burden. Time stands still for you. You perceive time differently; you don't experience it in as real a way as you normally do. 'What?! Summer is already over? I didn't even notice...' would be a typical statement.

Step 5: The Arm-Length Test

1. Stand up and let your arms hang loosely at your sides. Relax your shoulders and arms.

2. Now bring your hands together in a relaxed manner in front of your body, right at its centre. Turn the backs of your hands outward, so you can use your thumbnails as a measuring tool. When you are in balance, your thumbs are at the same height.

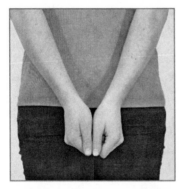

Arm-length test: 'yes', or balance

3. Bring your arms back to the sides of your body and remember to apply spherical vision.

4. Say 'yes', and once more bring your arms together in front of your body. Again, they will be equally long.

5. Relax your arms again and let them hang loosely at your sides.

6. Now say 'no' and bring your arms together in front of your body. This time, your thumbs will not be at the same height. There will be a difference in

length, except if you are caught in a state of rigidity (this will be explained in more detail in the next chapter). Your body says 'no'. It's stressed when it says something negative.

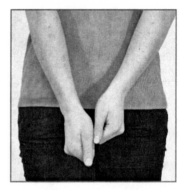

Arm-length test: 'No', or stress

7. Now practise this once more with your eyes closed. I often close my eyes when I want to sense something, as one can often see better this way.

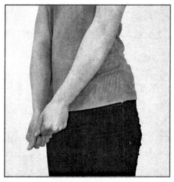

Arm-length test: position of both arms

At the beginning, the difference in the length of your arms during testing can often be fairly small: 1–3 cm (0.5–1.5 in). The more relaxed you become, and the more you practise, the larger it will be. Even differences of 10 cm (about 4 in) are not uncommon. Just relax, and your answers will be totally clear.

With time, it will no longer matter to you how your thumbs respond, because you will trust your body. You will have become a perfect tester.

In this way, you can talk to your subconscious through your body:

– Think of something positive and your arms will be of equal length.

– Think of something negative and the length of your arms will differ.

And your stress and lie detector is always with you.

TESTING: INITIAL SITUATIONS

Regular test

- When you say 'yes' and test, your arms are equally long.

- When you say 'no' and test, the length of your arms differs.

You are able to test!

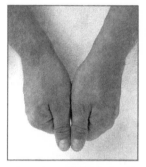

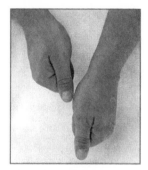

Arm-length test: 'yes', or balance

Arm-length test: 'no', or stress

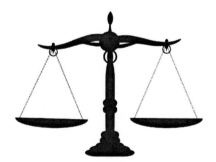

Scale in balance

Initial stress

*   With a 'yes', the length of your arms differs. You are out of balance. One side of your scale already has a weight on it.

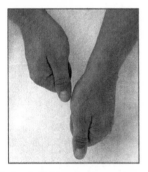

Arm-length test shows 'no', or stress response, with 'yes' statement

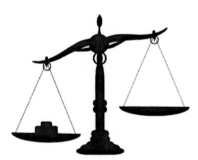

Scale out of balance

- With 'no', you are now adding a weight on the other side. The scale looks like it's balanced, although there are weights on both sides. For those of you who are more mathematically inclined: two 'no's equal one 'yes'.

The first thing to do is treat yourself!

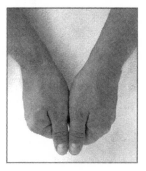

*Arm-length test shows what seems to be a 'yes',
or balance, with 'no' statement*

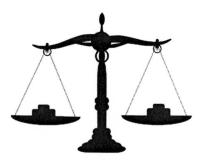

Scale with initial stress and 'no' statement

Blockage or rigidity

- You are frozen! Either in balance or in stress.

- Your arms no longer respond when you say 'yes' or 'no'. They remain the same – either equally long, or their length differs.

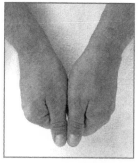
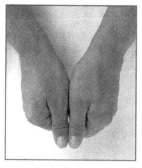

Arm-length test shows 'yes', or balance, with 'yes' statement

Arm-length test shows 'yes', or balance, with 'no' statement

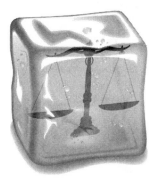

Shock frozen in balance

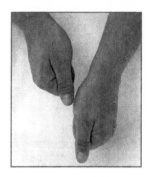 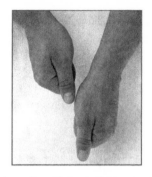

Arm-length test shows 'no', or stress response, with 'yes' statement

Arm-length test shows 'no', or stress response, with 'no' statement

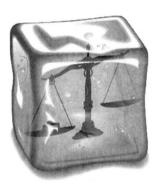

Shock frozen in stress

The first thing to do is treat yourself!

INITIAL STRESS AND STATE OF RIGIDITY: TREATING YOURSELF

There is always a remedy.

If you take the right thing, or just imagine it, your stress or blockage goes away.

You always have the right remedy around. Trust yourself.

Here are some remedies and ways to support healing:

- Drinking water

- Changing the colour of your clothes

- Imagining beautiful situations or colours

- Listening to music

- Speaking the truth

- Meditating

- Practising yoga

- Affirmations

- Prayers

- Painting

- Taking a shower

- Smelling flowers

- Drinking herbal teas

- Dancing

- Meditating with crystals

- Using Bach flower essences or homeopathy

- Going for a walk

You could also treat yourself with *Innerwise®: The Complete Healing System*

If you have the *Innerwise* card deck, imagine being balanced again and draw 1 to 5 healing cards, trusting your intuition. This re-establishes your balance. Now you are open again and able to continue testing as you would normally do. Place the healing cards in your hands and let them work. Take a few minutes to meditate with them. Then you can transfer them into your amulet.

When you have finished, your arms will be equally long when you say 'yes'; and when you say 'no', their lengths will differ. You are back in life.

WHAT CAN THE ARM-LENGTH TEST SHOW?

The arm-length test can do more than just show a 'yes' or 'no'. It can also express:

– A small no, or low stress

– A big no, or high stress

And it can reveal:

– Panic and allergies

The following images show all these possible scenarios:

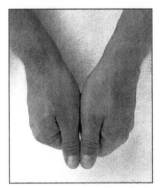

Arm-length test: 'yes', or balance

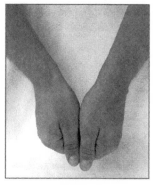

Arm-length test: small 'no', or low stress

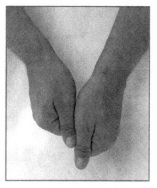

Arm-length test: medium 'no' or stress

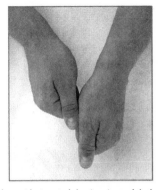

Arm-length test: big 'no', or high stress

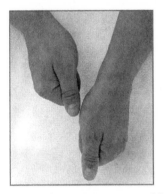

Arm-length test: huge 'no', or very high stress

Allergy or Panic

The difference in arm length will keep increasing as you repeat the testing several times in a row. The cause can be an allergy or an emotional panic.

– It's an **allergy** if you are testing food, a shampoo, a dental filling or any other material or substance to which you might have an allergic reaction.

– It's **panic** if you are thinking of a situation that causes a panic reaction in you.

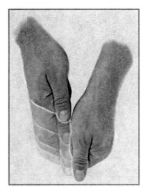

Arm-length test: allergy or panic response

Yes/No or Balance/Stress

How do I assess the response of my arms? This depends on what you are testing:

– If you test statements such as 'I do...', equally long arms indicates '**Balance. This is good for me**.'

Arms differing in length, however, mean '**Stress. This is not good for me**.'

With such statements, you can already test reliably as a beginner.

– If you test statements such as 'Should I do...?' or 'Does ... harm me?', assessing the response of your arms depends entirely on how the question is phrased. The test can only reveal a '**yes' or 'no'**.

If it really harms you, your arms will be equally long. Your body says 'yes'.

Testing questions is an option **which I recommend to those who are already confident in using the test,** and who consider in advance what a 'yes' or 'no' response to that question means to them.

Assessing the Test Response

When testing statements:

- Equally long arms: **balance. This is good for me**.

- Arms differing in length: **stress. This is not good for me**.

When testing questions:

- Equally long arms: **yes, this is correct**.

- Arms differing in length: **no, this is false**.

WHAT SHOULD YOU NOT TEST?

We are not supposed to know some things because we are meant to experience them. This is why you may not test certain things. If you do, you will get meaningless answers.

Our experience is our fortune! This is why questions about the future can often not be tested. Similarly lottery numbers, as the winnings would lead us away from our path of life.

Testing other people without their consent is not allowed and would often be manipulative.

Testing in order to manipulate, such as to create dependencies, or to gain control or harm others will certainly entail an 'extra round of experience'. Here, life is very fair.

To be on the safe side, it's best to start with the following questions:

1. Am I allowed to ask this question?

2. Will I get a meaningful response?

With these two questions you can avoid meaningless answers that will lead you astray.

If you obtain a 'yes' to both questions, you can ask the question.

USING THE TEST WHEREVER YOU ARE

Now it's up to you to use the test as much as possible. Test while standing up, lying down or sitting, both with your eyes open and with your eyes closed.

It's like learning how to play the piano, only it takes much less time. The more you practise using the arm-length test, the more confidence you will have in the results. Keep practising the 'yes' and 'no'.

Just test simple things, such as which colour you should pick for your clothes today.

Simply say, 'Shall I wear...', and then use the test, Your arms will tell you, 'Yes, go ahead', or 'No! Are you crazy?'

The more open you are, and the higher your vibrational frequency, the larger the differences in arm length during testing.

It's similar to a windscreen wiper: the larger the surface that is cleaned by the wiper, the greater the clarity.

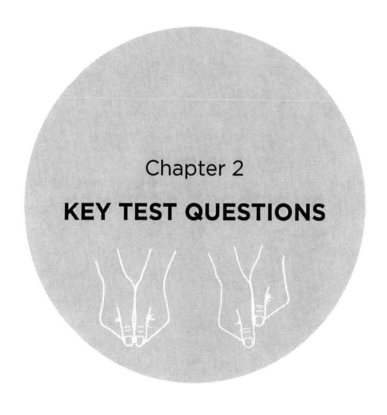

Chapter 2

KEY TEST QUESTIONS

LIFE IS LIKE CAKE BATTER

What does cake have to do with the course of our lives?

With cake batter, you can create any conceivable shape, yet it will always take the shape of the pan in which it's baked. The cake pan of our reality is our energy field. Our reality follows our energy field as it evolves.

However, our energy field is not a free, open and clear space; rather it's imprinted and shaped by our experiences, patterns and traumas. It's deformed, indented, imprisoned. It has rigid structures and has lost some parts. It was once free, unlimited and complete. That was at the very beginning of our Being. For most people, the energy field, and thus their reality's realm of possibilities to unfold, was already confined and indented when they were in their mother's womb.

And any life experience that we haven't yet fully accepted in love and peace keeps deforming our energy field.

Sometimes the energy field looks like a wrecked car, so reality has to be like that of a contortionist to find any free space left.

If you manage to free your energy field of limitations, you can heal and become whole again, complete and honest. You can exist as a person of integrity. Then you are once again free in creating your reality. And you can enjoy this unlimitedness.

To clear your energy field, you need the right tools, as words alone won't suffice. You will also not achieve this with mere willpower, nor through fighting or manipulation.

The access to our energy field is through the heart, and the subconscious, which is receptive to sounds, colours, frequencies and energies.

WHAT IS GOOD HEALTH?

Good health is harmony, which you can imagine as a beautifully curved sinusoid. With emotional or energetic stress, however, the beautiful sinusoid turns into a flatline. We enter a state of disharmony.

In this state, the body can no longer truly live, only survive. It tries everything to get out of this disharmony – be it a cold, diarrhoea, a headache, or sometimes even an accident. Whatever symptoms appear, the important thing at first is to create chaos. Chaos is the response to the state of rigidity, and it's precisely this chaos we call illness. Meanwhile, chaos bears the chance of healing; the real problem was the state of rigidity we were in previously.

Using the arm-length test, you can determine exactly when the state of harmony is starting to fade – you experience initial stress or rigidity when you test.

If you restore harmonious balance immediately, you can prevent chaos in most cases, or at least reduce its duration significantly.

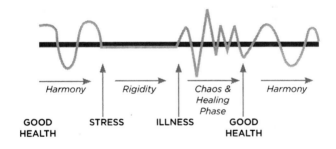

The cycle of illness and good health

A JOURNEY THROUGH TIME

This is a way to test where a certain problem or disharmony really originated. Many things go back further than we think.

A woman went on a trip for a few days. While she was staying with her girlfriend, she sounded happy and full of energy on the phone. Then she took the train back home. The journey lasted seven hours and, when talking to her on the phone while she was still on the train, her voice already sounded subdued and exhausted.

When she arrived home, the woman was in a complete state of rigidity. Her life energy was at 30 per cent. She assumed that the train ride hadn't been good for her. The arm-length test showed that the lengths of her arms differed, with no change between 'yes' and 'no'. The woman was caught in a state of rigidity.

Then, going back in time in her mind, she imagined different points in time.

Yesterday evening around 6 p.m.: the result of the arm-length test was normal. Today at 8 a.m., before taking the train: she was in a state of rigidity. Yesterday evening at 9 p.m.: regular test result. 10 p.m.: rigidity.

Then it dawned on her. She had watched a horror movie with her girlfriend and it had scared her.

The journey through time quickly revealed the true source of the rigidity. The train had not been the problem.

With a journey through time it's possible to travel back many years.

The heart of a 40-year-old man shows stress:

– Heart at 30 years: stress.

– Heart at 20 years: no stress.

– Heart at 21 years: stress.

And the answer already bubbles out of his mouth:

'That was when my girlfriend left me, and it took me years to get over it.'

It's like taking an elevator through time. No information about the past has been lost. You only need to ask and retrieve it.

I had a 65-year-old patient who, for the previous 12 weeks, had been having problems again with her stomach and bladder; she also had trouble sleeping, and the sniffles. Using the arm-length test, I'd tested that the causes of these symptoms dated from the age of 14. Then she told me that at the age of 14, she had contracted polio. She had to spend many weeks in the hospital, isolated behind glass.

After that, she needed two years in order to be able to move again more or less normally. She managed, except for her left arm, which remained paralysed. Three months ago she went on holiday. In her hotel room, the bathtub was set up in exactly the opposite way to her home. For this reason, she couldn't help herself with the paralysed arm, and all the bad polio-related memories came back... together with a lot of tears. Since then, she had been stuck in a panic reaction and had fallen ill.

I love this test! I would never have found out how all of this was connected. Within just five minutes, I managed to restore her balance, enabling all her symptoms to disappear.

100% LIFE ENERGY: GO GET IT!

Life energy is the magic force we receive as a gift from life.

It has many names: vitality, *prana*, *qi*, *orgon*, life force or simply life energy.

What's special about is that no device can measure it, no biophysicist is able to patent it, and it's not described in any school book for children. Yet everybody knows about it.

Most people only start appreciating it once they've lost it. Then they feel drained, tired, lacking strength, no longer able to perform, and they find excuses for this state, such as 'I'm getting old.' This is not true. There are children who have lost almost all their life energy, and there are 90-year-olds whose batteries are almost full.

When you lack energy, life becomes agony. All that's left is to stick it out. If, however, as an adult you feel 20 years younger than you actually are, you have plenty of life energy.

But if you feel as old as you are, or even older, then it's time to recharge your batteries.

Which angel do you feel like being?

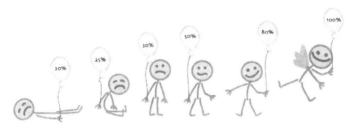

Life energy angels

63

And which angel do you feel you are right now?

Ranging from zero to 100 per cent, how much life energy do you have?

Or, in more casual terms, with 0 per cent you are pushing up daisies and with 100 per cent you are flying.

Find the answer within you; trust your intuition.

I've tested the life energy of thousands of patients and from this data I drew up a life energy list.

The Life Energy Scale

100 per cent: it's like flying, or like being newly in love.

80 per cent: able to perform at full capacity, reaching your goals.

70 per cent: able to perform at normal capacity; you've been better.

50 per cent: hanging in there, but it's no fun anymore.

40 per cent: able to perform for four to six hours.

30 per cent: exhausted after two hours of work; crying more frequently.

25 per cent: deep exhaustion; nothing matters anymore.

20 per cent: the batteries are empty.

You can use the arm-length test to gauge your life energy level yourself.

It's really easy. Just as if you wanted to ask the following questions about a water bottle: 'Is there any water here?' Answer: 'yes'.

A bit higher: 'Is there any water here?' Response: 'yes'.

And still a bit higher: 'Is there any water here?' Response: 'no'.

Of course, you enquire slightly differently.

Say:

'My life energy is 50 per cent.'

Then test using your arms. If the response is 'yes', your thumbs will be at the same height.

Then say:

'My life energy is 60 per cent.'

Continue until you have determined the exact value.

If you receive a 'no' response at 70 per cent, for example, the level of your life energy is between 60 and 70 per cent.

If you get a 'no' at 50 per cent, i.e. your thumbs are not at the same height, then continue asking about 40 per cent. Keep reducing the percentage until your arms respond with a 'yes' and you have determined the value.

Perhaps you find out that your level of life energy is 30 per cent and you feel depressed. You can see yourself as a victim: 'I have only 30 per cent. Poor me! Please give me happy pills.'

Or you can grow up and ask yourself where the missing 70 per cent is.

It hasn't disappeared. There is always 100 per cent. The question is merely how you use this 100 per cent.

You can use it for yourself and your life path. Then it's life energy. And you can use it against yourself. Then it's destructive energy; that is, your compromises and lies.

Tough luck: by 'being a victim' you won't get any further than the happy pills, and you'll become a drug addict of the pharmaceutical industry.

A better way is to grow up and take responsibility for your life. Put an end to all the compromises you've been making that eat up your energy, and change your life. Regain your energy. You are worth it because your soul is beautiful and lovable!

Now you know how much energy you are using for yourself as life energy. The energy missing from the full 100 per cent is energy you are using against yourself. These are your compromises. With those, you are destroying yourself.

I AM MYSELF: 'I AM I'

- **I am (first name).**

- **I am living my own life and not somebody else's**.

When I test whether I am myself and say, 'I am I', my arms should remain equally long, i.e. respond with 'yes'.

About half of the readers of this book will not have this response – their response will be 'no'. If you are not you, who are you? Don't be surprised, this can happen. It can happen in the best families... we drift off our paths and try to live somebody else's life.

There are only two reasons for not having our own identities, and why testing 'I am I' yields a 'no' response.

1. We think we have to bear the burden for other people and help carry their problems; then we have what's commonly referred to as the 'helper syndrome'. Yet everyone is allowed to, or should be able to, gain his or her own experiences. We don't want to deprive anybody of his or her right to make a decision, do we?

2. There is the big world of manipulation: In his book *The Celestine Prophecy*, James Redfield described perfectly how we try to steal energy from other people. A very popular way to set up this energy pipeline is to give somebody another identity. This doesn't usually happen consciously, of course, but this is no excuse. And the other side allowed this energy-sucking to happen.

You know this feeling: you feel good, you are doing just fine. Then you meet somebody and you feel like a totally different person. Your good mood is gone, your energy is drained, your voice has changed and your face looks different – as if you were not yourself anymore.

If you then test using the arm-length test and say, 'I am I', you will get a 'no' response: the length of your arms will differ. The other person has stolen your energy, your identity.

Now, you should quickly help yourself. If you want to walk your own path in life, you need your own identity back.

I AM HEALTHY

- I'm free from infections.

- I'm free from allergies.

- I'm free from deficiencies.

- My organs are in harmony.

- My breath is free.

- My body is in balance.

I AM HAPPY

- I am happy.

- I breathe freely, my eyes are shining, I dance through life.

I AM HONEST WITH MYSELF AND OTHERS

- I am honest.

- I say what I think and feel, regardless of the consequences.

I AM READY TO CHANGE

- I am ready to change EVERYTHING to live a healthy and happy life.

Your current state is the result of your way of life. If you are not happy with this situation, you have to be ready to change your life without any concern.

Or you continue suffering. You have the choice.

I NOURISH MYSELF IN HEALTHY WAYS

- I'm nourished on all levels: on the emotional, energetic, spiritual, mental and physical levels.

Think about what nourishes you. What nourishes your heart, your brain, your cells, your longing for touch? We are nourished by all that we eat, drink, see, feel, hear, dream, think or touch.

Only when we understand it in this way can a diet really make sense.

What does a diet mean for you?

- To avoid watching TV and reading the newspaper?

- To free your home from everything that you don't really need?

- To meditate? To stay silent?

- To give up anger, fury, rage and resentment?

- To focus on what's important right now?

- To do without coffee, alcohol and chocolate?

- Or simply to eat less?

I TAKE GOOD CARE OF MYSELF

• I cleanse myself of any poisons in my life: negative thoughts, bitter feelings, negative energies, painful memories, toxic chemicals, heavy metals in my mouth, dishonest life situations.

What was the greatest poison in your life? This also includes heavy metals and chemicals. Most people answer this question differently:

Fear, guilt, disappointment, spiritual trauma, having felt unloved... these are the most frequent replies.

I LOVE MYSELF

- I love what I was, what I am and what I will be.

There are no mistakes, just experiences.

- I'm ready to open my heart and give up my protection. I'm ready to give and receive love.

I allow myself to be vulnerable again.

I AM WORTH IT

- I am worth being healthy, happy, loved, successful...

I AM SELF-RESPONSIBLE

- I don't use anybody for my purposes, nor do I allow anybody to use me.

- I take responsibility for my life.

- I trust other people to take responsibility for their own lives.

CHECKLIST PRIOR TO EACH TEST

1. Use spherical vision.

2. Say 'yes' and test: your (and the test subject's) arms should be equally long.

3. Say 'no' and test: your (and the test subject's) arms should differ in length.

4. Test if you are allowed to test this question when it concerns the future or other people: 'Am I allowed to ask this question?' 'Will I receive a meaningful response?'

Chapter 3

USING THE ARM-LENGTH TEST THROUGHOUT THE DAY

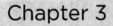

WHAT SHOULD I WEAR TODAY?

A shirt or a t-shirt? A skirt or trousers? Which clothes fit the weather? In which colour do I feel good today?

Colours are also frequencies and they can support or balance but also irritate us.

Stand in front of your wardrobe and think of the day and what's waiting for you. Imagine wearing this or that. And then test your body's response.

Today I will wear...

It takes trust in the answer, as the following episodes show.

Choosing my clothes

We wanted to go to a big event and, as usual, 'I didn't have anything to wear.' The test was supposed to help me choose the right clothes, but I didn't like the answer. The test kept showing stress, although the colour of the sweater suited me perfectly and concealed all my chubby parts. I decided to wear it regardless, a decision I regretted within minutes of entering the hall. It was terribly warm in there, and I had decided to wear a beautiful turtleneck that was guaranteed to cause me STRESS.

Monika F., teacher

Which t-shirt should I wear today?

When I get up in the morning and don't really know what to wear, and start having doubts, the arm-length test quickly helps me choose what suits me best that day. Using the arm-length test, I ask which clothes I should wear today. And so far I have been very happy with the result, as are those around me.

Bianca L., student

WHAT FOODS WILL HELP ME FEEL GOOD TODAY?

Just because something *tastes* good to you doesn't mean that it *is* good for you. You could have a burning desire for a certain food or drink although you are allergic to it.

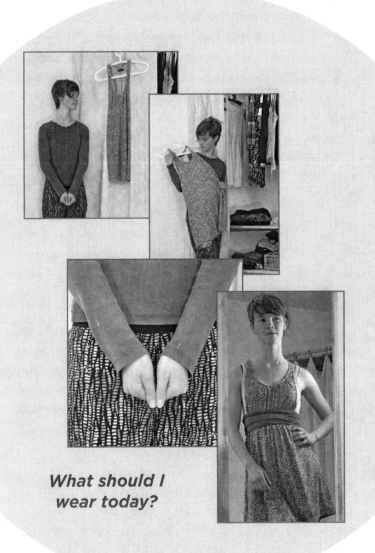

What should I wear today?

Why? Because your body produces stress hormones when you have that food or drink. These hormones give you a little high – basically, it's hormone doping. Just like jogging, when the body produces its own happy hormones (endorphins).

We react to food in three different ways. We can tolerate or not tolerate certain foods, or we can be allergic to them. And we can need or not need certain foods.

The arm-length test indicates an allergic reaction when the difference in arm length keeps increasing as you test several times in a row.

The most common food allergies are to cow's milk protein, chicken protein, wheat, colourants and preservatives. Allergic symptoms don't always appear immediately, nor are they directly visible. Rather, they can become apparent in a more hidden way as an inflammation of the gum tissue, a middle ear infection, asthma, the sniffles, fatigue, poor concentration, intestinal inflammation, smelly armpit perspiration or edemas.

If you are allergic to milk protein, bear in mind that the actual allergen is cow protein. This includes steak, milk, curd, butter, cheese, yoghurt, chocolate, potato crisps... yes, check out the ingredients. You will simply have to avoid anything made from the cow. Alternatively, you can resort to sheep and goat products.

Most people who have stopped consuming the food they are allergic to, and have, so to speak, gone through a withdrawal, develop a natural nausea to this food.

Test all the food that you like to eat or drink.
Test all the products in your fridge.

Learn to test everything already at the supermarket *before* you spend money on food products that you or your family can't tolerate.

Stand in front of the food products and imagine eating or drinking them. Then test them.

Or say:

- I eat...

- I drink...

- I can tolerate it!

- My family can tolerate it!

- It's good for everybody in my family!

- I need it.

- It's good for me.

Chocolate-hazelnut spread

My 10-year-old daughter attended the Innerwise children's workshop. During testing she thought about checking out her favourite food, a super-sweet chocolate-hazelnut spread. She tested stress. She got quite huffy and said, 'But I'll keep eating it anyway.' I decided not to go there and didn't say anything. A few days later, she left for camp. When she returned she told me proudly: 'They also had a chocolate-hazelnut spread there but I didn't eat any the whole week because it's not good for me.'

Eva R., educator

GOING SHOPPING

Should I do my shopping in this supermarket, or in the organic store instead?

In front of the cheese shelf:

• Imagine eating a particular cheese, and test.

Or ask:

• Do I tolerate this cheese?

• Do I like this cheese?

• Does my partner like this cheese?

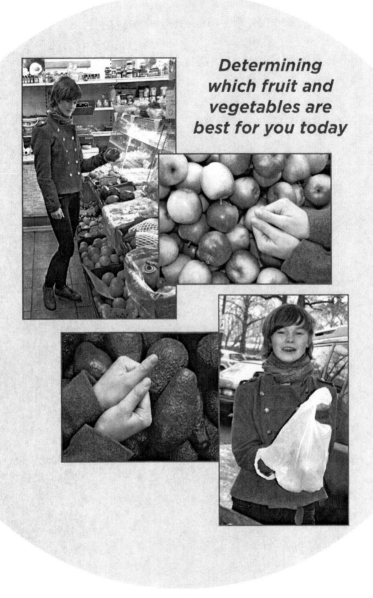

Determining which fruit and vegetables are best for you today

When choosing fruit or vegetables:

- Are certain fruit and vegetables good for me today?

- This one?

- Or will this one be best?

At the wine shelf:

- Is there any wine that is OK for me?

- On this shelf?

- Back there?

When choosing the detergent:

- Does my whole family tolerate this detergent?

- Do we tolerate the dishwasher tabs?

Some chemicals that can be toxic or cause an allergic reaction always remain on the dishes. In the future, simply test everything before you buy it. You and your family will have many fewer stomach aches and far fewer problems with food allergies.

Incidentally, the best thing to do in case of middle ear infections, asthma or intestinal problems is to leave out all dairy products, because there is often an intolerance to cow's milk protein behind this.

In case of smelly sweat, you should test coffee and black and green tea, as well as chocolate. Many people are not able to eliminate the alkaloids that act as stimulants in these products via the kidneys or the liver. So they are released through the skin as smelly sweat.

Choosing the right birthday present

We were invited to a birthday party at a new friend's house, and we didn't yet know her likes and dislikes. In such a situation it's difficult to find a fitting present. We love angel figurines, so we tested if she would also enjoy receiving one as a present. The arm-length response was 'no'. We then bought another gift that didn't indicate any stress. At the birthday party, we noticed that she was very happy with the present that had tested positive. Using the arm-length test, we then also tested whether her joy was honest, and it was. When we chatted about the idea of offering an angel as a gift, she confirmed that they didn't mean anything to her and that she wouldn't like to receive them as a present.

Bettina P., business economist

On a shopping tour

When we go shopping for clothes and my daughter doesn't always get all that she wants, she promptly suggests: 'Hey Mum, let's test if we shouldn't buy that one, too.'

Juliane P., teacher

WHICH ROUTE SHOULD I TAKE?

Before I take the car to go anywhere, I always test if I will arrive safely. Sometimes I get a 'no' for an answer. I don't drive off before I have clarified why. It can be that I should take a different route, or that I still have something important to do before leaving.

Should I take this route (or that one)?

Will I arrive safely and without having an accident?

Finding the right route

We were in Cyprus driving our rental car on a well-built road. Suddenly, I had a bad feeling which was confirmed by the arm-length test. I asked my husband to turn right into a side road immediately. It was the original and pretty demanding road connecting us back to the new route. There, I understood the alleged reason for my bad feeling. There had just been an accident on the main road involving three cars and it was now closed.

Heidrun J., bookseller

Riding your bike accident-free

Last week, I was eager to take my bike into town. I knew I would find just the right present for my grandchild in a certain store. Yet I had a very bad feeling, and the arm-length test confirmed that there could possibly be an accident. On the way, suddenly an older man opened the driver's door of his parked car. Only the fact that I kept a larger distance than usual to the parked cars I passed avoided a collision.

Anette Sch., retiree

GPS or the arm-length test – which is right?

I was driving from Ulm to Munich when, shortly before entering the highway, I suddenly heard the following GPS announcement: 'The route is being recalculated due to traffic information update.' This meant not taking the highway but a country road. Since I was under time pressure, I asked my arms, and they clearly said: 'Continue on the highway as planned.'

I trusted the result, already expecting the friendly voice from the GPS telling me: 'Idiot! I just told you to take another route.' But it didn't and the traffic jam didn't materialize either. And I was in Munich on time.

Eric G., programmer

SEEK AND FIND

The following examples speak for themselves.

Finding the right tool

I needed to look for a certain tool in my brother's workshop. Unfortunately, he wasn't reachable, so I couldn't ask him directly where he kept it. I imagined the tool and with the arm-length test, I checked out in which direction I should search the rooms of his workshop.

The workshop is really big and has lots of different tools and equipment, yet it didn't take me long to find the tool.

Jörg E., long-haul truck driver

Finding a bathing suit in the chaos

The arm-length test also helps when facing chaos. My bathing suit had got lost in the depths of my wardrobe. So I stood in front of my wardrobe and asked, 'Where should I look for it?' On the first three shelves, the response indicated stress, and on the fourth one it was balanced. The bathing suit was on the fourth shelf, behind a large pile of sweaters. And I had saved myself a great deal of stress!

Yvonne Z., saleswoman

Looking for mushrooms in the forest

It was a beautiful Sunday in summer and I felt it was the right time to go to the forest to look for edible mushrooms. We walked together to the nearby forest. To determine where to go and which direction to take, we used the arm-length test. We didn't yet know of any specific area in the forest where we could find edible mushrooms. Our focus was: 'We want to find a parasol or a giant puffball-type mushroom.' We were searching around, guided by the arm-length test, when we finally found a small puffball (it was a bit larger than my fist). We kept looking but couldn't find any more edible mushrooms in the area.

Later we found out that we hadn't asked the question correctly. That is to say, it makes a difference whether you are looking for one mushroom or a bag of mushrooms...

Jakob H., student

Finding a well

I can still remember when I was looking for the right place to dig a new well with iron-free water. With the help of my intuition, I had found it quickly; it didn't even take five minutes. But could this be true? The arm-length test said 'yes'. For one entire week, I verified the responses on a daily basis. The results were always the same, including the drilling depth. And the well-builders confirmed them all in their work.

Andreas F., fish farmer

EATING AT HOME OR EATING OUT?

Eating at home or eating out? Simply test what's best for you today.

At home, you can go to the fridge and test all the food items. Or you can imagine the plate with the prepared dish and then ask your arms.

Of course, it could happen that suddenly, being a strict vegetarian, you would be allowed to have a bite of a chicken leg. But then you have an excuse: it was your arms that decided this...

Another time, the response could imply a few fasting days. Simply learn to trust your body again. It knows best what's good for it.

If you want to eat out, use the menu to test the right dish for you today.

- Is the best food for me today on this page, or on that page?

- Is it...?

In this way, your ordering will be quick and right to the point!

Tasty and healthy – which lunch menu is best for me today?

At the canteen at work, we can choose from three menus and a small dish for lunch. Often, deciding what to eat is not that easy. Especially when several of the menus look good to me. I then ask myself and test which menu I can tolerate best today. Since

I've started doing this, it's usually a good choice and I can digest the dish very well. At times, I don't go with the recommendation that my arm-length test shows me. Then it often happens that I don't digest the dish that well.

Felix Sch., church employee

Tea of the day

My daughter was preparing some tea for herself and asked me if I also wanted some, and which one I preferred. I told her 'whichever', and that she should pick one. Then she asked me to come to the kitchen and said to me, 'Hey, Mum, let's test which one would be good for you.' And so I had the tea that fitted me perfectly that day.

Birgit R., nurse

COOKING WITH THE MICROWAVE

One of my mother's girlfriends, a teacher of home economics, always used to say: 'If you love your husband, you don't use the microwave for cooking unless you are already looking forward to being a widow.'

I also don't eat or drink anything in restaurants that has been heated up in a microwave, because my stomach doesn't tolerate it.

Test for yourself. Take three glasses of water. Fill one up with tap water; boil the water for the other in an electric kettle or on the stove, and heat up the water for the third glass in a microwave. Then, let them all cool down to the same temperature and test the different glasses:

- Imagine drinking these glasses of water and test.

Or ask yourself:

- Is it good for me to drink this water?

Since all food contains water, you can apply the water test results to any other food as well.

DELICIOUS COOKING WITHOUT A RECIPE

I've been cooking for years without a cookbook. I test the food combination, the ingredients, spices and cooking times... and my family likes it!

Dad's recipe-free cooking

My dad cooks the most delicious meals, without any recipe. He always comes up with them himself, or more precisely, he tests them. He stands in front of the fridge and tests what fits us best on that day. Then, everything flies wildly into the pot. The spice shelf descends on the food via the arm-length test, and the end result is almost always simply delicious!

Hannah A., student

RESTFUL SLEEP

We spend one third of our lives sleeping, so we should also enjoy this time.

You fall asleep within a few minutes and sleep through the night. In the morning, you wake up with a clear mind, free of pain and well-rested. Congratulations! Unfortunately, for most people it's not like that.

- Imagine lying in your bed for the whole night and test with your arms.

If there is a difference in arm length, the place where you sleep is not good for you. It's not really possible to have a relaxed and restful sleep there.

- Now imagine again lying in your bed for the whole night. Then imagine there is no power in the whole building, nor in the power cables outside your window, if there are any.

If your arms are now equally long, the source of your problem is electrosmog.

If there is still a difference in arm length, your problem is geopathology; or it bears the name of your partner with whom you share the bed (which is rarely the case).

- So... imagine once more... your partner doesn't lie there or another partner lies there...

If your arms are equally long now, it's time to think about whether you want to save this partnership or not.

But let's get to what's most frequently the source of the problem: geopathology.

Imagine sleeping in a different place, moving the bed or sleeping in a different room.

If your arms are equally long now, great! Change the place where you sleep – now, tonight – to finally have a good night's sleep again.

However, it can take a few days to adjust. Hang in there!

Geopathological interference zones are harmful to us because they interfere with our cell metabolism, cause tissue acidification and an increase in muscle tension. This leads to back pain.

If you are sleeping in such a zone (cats love such spots but dogs would never sleep there), you will never get rid of your back pain. But now you can test all of this yourself with your arms.

It's a bit more challenging with electrosmog. This applies if, during testing, the arms become equally long when you imagine there is no power. The typical symptoms are trouble falling asleep and urination at night. You don't wake up with a clear mind in the morning. Only taking a cold shower and/or a coffee helps you start your day in a fairly bearable way.

This is caused by a disturbed regulatory hormone production in the pineal and pituitary glands. Since our bodies contains water, electric current flows through them when we are in an AC electric field. As a result, the pineal and pituitary glands become lazy, because AC voltage is misinterpreted as daylight.

The glands think they don't have to work, because the pineal gland works at night and the pituitary gland always waits for its instructions.

With the body lacking regulatory hormones, you feel as if you've been beaten up instead of well rested in the morning. The most common cause is the AC electric fields of the electric cables attached to your bedside light or radio alarm clock, or inside the wall.

You can easily measure the harmful effects with a measuring device. So-called coupling measurements gauge the AC voltage in the human body. Here, 0.1 volts are considered the upper limit for reasonably harmful effects. I recommend the following measures:

1. Remove all extension cords near your bed, i.e. within 2 m (about 6.5 feet).

2. For two weeks, turn off the circuit breakers while you sleep. If the quality of your sleep improves tangibly, commission an electrician who knows how to set up electrical installations according to building biology to take care of the problem.

3. Clear away the harmful effects through protective shielding. Here, conductive material is installed and grounded between the voltage source and the place where you sleep, such as the E-Cover product that I developed.

Even my husband trusts the test now

Having worked with Innerwise for a number of years, I can hardly imagine life without it. I use it in my everyday life, for instance, when I go shopping. Even my husband now trusts the arm-length test in many situations.

This is a short overview of concrete questions:

– Do we like this food?

– Do I tolerate this food? (I once had a food allergy.)

– Will my guests like this food?

– Will the gift I picked out bring joy to its recipient?

– Will he like these flowers?

– Will these clothes fit my grandchild (who's not here)?

– Do I feel stress when buying a specific product?

All information I receive simply allows me to feel more confident and sure of myself.

By using Innerwise more and more often, my intuitive abilities also improved tangibly with time, so that I don't need to use the arm-length test anymore. Today, I can rely perfectly well on my feelings.

Anna T., retiree

Chapter 4

THE ARM-LENGTH TEST IN ALL LIFE SITUATIONS

THE ARM-LENGTH TEST FOR HEALTH

From Conception to Birth and Infancy

Hoping to Conceive

Most couples hoping to conceive reveal stress during the arm-length test when they imagine that the partner has become pregnant, or that they already have a child. It's a subconscious stress.

If this stress is removed, the woman usually gets pregnant within a month.

I am Pregnant!

Our arms are faster than any test strips can be. Just bear in mind that women get pregnant much more often than they know, since 60 to 70 per cent of all fertilized egg cells don't survive the first two to three weeks.

You're going to have a baby

With our last child, my five-year-old daughter said to my partner on the 12th day after conception: 'You're pregnant. You're going to have a baby, I can see it.' I had gathered this based on what the arm-length test had revealed to me, but of course, clairvoyant children are even better at this.

Uwe A., author

During Pregnancy

Is the child in the womb doing well? Does it need anything? Does the mother feel healthy, safe and secure? You can test this easily.

The need for vitamins, minerals, more rest; or the wish for a bouquet of flowers, a few days of holiday or a good talk... you can easily test all this within seconds. And there's no need to spend a long time searching for the cause of the discontent.

Birth and Infancy

During this time, many people in both of the partners' environments will gladly and often give advice based on their experience. And you might hear that 'things have always been done this way'.

Yet deep inside, you have some doubts as to whether all this well-meant advice is also good for you. For this reason, test everything and listen to the response you receive, even if nobody understands why.

If, for instance, neither of you want to have any visitors during the first few weeks after your child is born, then stand by your feeling. Nobody can make demands on you.

Test what's good for the baby and act accordingly.

Let the baby sleep together with you in your bed, carry it around, always let it feel close to you. Breastfeed your baby whenever it wants to.

Let your baby feel the comfort, safety and security it needs as it starts out in life.

The heart talks

The arm-length test has been a precious and integral part of my everyday life for many years. It's my body giving a physical voice to my subconscious. Expressing my heart's truth, it supports me in all questions and decisions when I need clarity on:

– What's really going on with me or in a particular situation.

– What something is really about.

– What's good for me and what isn't.

– What's the best decision or choice now, in tune with everything that is.

This can concern very basic things like what to eat or drink, or a purchase, as well as personal issues, relationships, my environment, animals, plants, work, my profession and my calling, or various activities, such as writing.

The arm-length is also a wonderful tool when doing energy work with others.

Irina P., translator

Testing Contraceptives

Only about 10 per cent of all women tolerate their contraceptive pill without any side effects. In contrast, 90 per cent of all women complain about side effects. The liver, breasts and veins can fall ill. Loss of libido plays a major role as well. But there are also many cases of intolerance with IUDs, condoms, gels, etc.

When testing contraceptives, bear in mind not to test the pill or IUD just for the current moment, as often the long-term intake is the cause of the problem.

- Do I tolerate the contraceptive pill?

- Do I tolerate it when I take it for several months?

- Do I tolerate it when I take it for years?

- Does my partner also tolerate this condom?

If you don't tolerate the prescribed pill, the best thing to do is go see your gynaecologist, stand in front of their pharmaceutical samples and test them.

Be brave, it's about your body! And then you can lend your doctor this book.

Intuition communicating through my arms

I cannot imagine life without feeling connected to my intuition. Being connected to one's intuition means for me to be connected to myself and to my higher self, to life, to the collective consciousness, and to be able to feel and experience life in unimagined depth and abundance. It allows me to sense and perceive other people, the environment and situations from a much higher perspective of understanding. For me, it creates the essential basis for living an authentic life; facing life with an open heart while remaining true to myself and for bringing this in tune with mind and reason.

It enables me to let go more and more and to want to control less. It helps me live in the flow. 'For the greatest benefit of all' serves as the guiding motto for making decisions accordingly. Thanks to my intuition, I can better see and understand the signs of life and feel and benefit from the power and potential of the moment more clearly and deeply.

The arm-length test helps me get to the bottom of what is actively, but still subconsciously, influencing me; it allows me to test it and grasp it. With time, my sensing and reaction have become ever more fine-tuned. I already sense the shift in tension in my body at a very fine level. This has changed my life fundamentally, and I'm deeply grateful for the invaluable support this method offers to me.

Irina P., translator

Vaccinations: Yes or No?

Vaccinations can be useful, but about 80 per cent of all vaccinated people experience vaccine-related damage.

Nobody gets six serious diseases at the same time, yet this is what we expect our babies to deal with. Combination vaccines contain components against six diseases in one: tetanus, diphtheria, whooping cough, polio, *Haemophilus influenzae* infection and hepatitis

B. With the vaccines come protein particles, antibiotics, formaldehyde, preservatives and heavy metals that are also injected into the body.

It's very important to test which vaccines by which manufacturer are tolerated in which combination. This can be done by therapists who are also medical doctors and know how to use the testing methods. Ask your doctor to test the vaccines before applying them; if he or she can't do that, go to a doctor who can and wants to do it.

It's also necessary to test the right timing of a vaccination; this cannot be predetermined by a calendar based on statistical calculations. Take all this into account and do the testing, then you can have your child vaccinated.

I can do it myself

For me, using the arm-length test was the first step on the path to self-determination and self-responsibility. At a doctor's practice, I had already experienced kinesiological testing via my right arm (food intolerance). But it wasn't until I attended your seminar that I realized I was also able to test myself, without the help of a medical doctor.

What followed was an interplay between euphoria and disenchantment. It took some time until I realized that from my perspective, the arm-length test only reveals reliable information when I remain true to myself, without the willpower of my ego. As soon as the mind chatter interferes, it's over. Even today.

Of course, self-confidence also plays a major role here. The less self-confidence there is, the faster questioning will set in from the outside. If the answer is clear, it takes trust and courage to make the decision and implement it. When I lacked trust and confidence, I engaged in evasive manoeuvres that went nowhere until I had reached the 'zero point' again. Then, if I didn't know what to do anymore, I remembered the test and was able to reorient myself.

What's also important to me is the realization that, with the arm-length test, I learned to trust my own physical reactions and perceptions. The 'yes' or 'no' response provides the confirmation. For instance, when I walk by my fishponds and I sense how my fish are doing, and I'm able to act accordingly.

Andreas F., fish farmer

Do I Need Vitamin Pills?

Since food is often no longer produced in good soil and of a high quality, vitamin supplements are sometimes needed for us to stay healthy in spite of the high stress levels and adverse influences of our times.

Vitamin C is recommended to boost the immune system, vitamin B to enhance the nervous system, and zinc against inflammations and as a multi-purpose pill for and against everything. I recommend you test these supplements before taking them, asking the following questions:

- Do I need... ?

- Do I tolerate... ?

And if you receive a positive answer to both:

- For how many days do I need to take... ?

- How many times a day do I need to take... ?

- What dose should I take?

From the Health Check-up to Self-healing

Our organs have different levels: the spiritual, energetic, emotional, mental and structural (organic) levels. Any illness starts in the subconscious, often as an imbalance on the energetic or emotional level.

Sooner or later, the disturbance reaches the organic level if the underlying issues are not resolved. Conventional medicine calls this 'illness'. At some point, a broken heart becomes a weak heart; with time, the laboratory values of a liver eaten up by anger will show pathological changes.

- I want to get healthy.

- I still need my illness for a reason.

- The cause of my illness is spiritual.

- The cause of my illness is energetic.

- The cause of my illness is emotional.

- The cause of my illness is mental.

- The cause of my illness is biochemical.

- The cause of my illness is organic.

- My illness is related to... (issues, people, decisions).

- I can heal myself.

- What helps me is...

- To heal, I need to change...

You can also touch the organ. For example, put your hand on the liver or the heart and test if it causes a stress response in your arms. If so, the organ has a problem on one of the aforementioned levels. With the liver, the cause can be alcohol, but frequently it's swallowed anger. As for the heart, a vessel could cause a problem, yet often the heart is broken. With the lungs, it's mostly unshed tears, and kidneys frequently reflect the distress of heavy losses in our lives.

Each organ can have a problem on the spiritual, energetic, emotional, mental, biochemical or organic level or on several levels.

If you lightly touch the liver and your arms indicate a difference in length, it means that your liver is stressed. Nothing more, nothing less. To find out on which level the liver is stressed, you can test the following:

- Liver on the structural level.

- Liver on the biochemical level.

- Liver on the mental level.

- Liver on the emotional level.

- Liver on the energetic level.

- Liver on the spiritual level.

The level causing a difference in arm length is where the problem lies.

Often, it's important to clarify since when there has been stress to find the source of a problem. Then it's easier to recognize how it's all connected.

If your heart shows stress, test if there was also stress five years ago.

If so, try six years ago, and so on, until you are at the point in time when the stress in your heart originated. It's almost always moments in your life that hurt when your body came out of balance.

If we are able to recognize an imbalance in time, we are usually also able to resolve it quite easily.

If there is a difference in arm length when you imagine being healthy again, you cannot get healthy. Your subconscious feels you need a different experience.

Then it's time to retune it. And you can test what this requires. It could be a number of different things or activities: drinking a specific herbal tea, having an honest conversation, writing and sending off a letter long overdue, making a decision, forgiving somebody, taking Bach flower essences, or something else.

You can also use *Innerwise®: The Complete Healing System* for this purpose. If you use it regularly to balance yourself, you will be able to avoid many illnesses.

Once you have found the remedy, your arms will be equally long when you imagine being healthy again.

When I get a cold...

Which rarely happens, because I test myself regularly with the arm-length test and take care of little irritations immediately, I quickly find a solution in my homeopathic home medical chest, or in my herb garden. And I haven't had to see my doctor in a long time.

Elvira Sch., tax official

Measuring blood sugar with the arm-length test

One day, I thought of testing my mother's blood-sugar level with the arm-length test immediately before measuring it with the blood glucose device, and to compare the results. The first measurement results I tested were a bit off the mark. When applying this test, it's necessary to be fully centred and very calm inside. After a stressful day at work, I didn't manage this.

Another approach came to mind. When testing the value, I imagined measuring the blood-sugar level using the measuring units of the device, so that the tested values I would obtain corresponded to these units. Keeping this present as I tested, I then took measurements using the arm-length test, and obtained, for instance, a value of 220 for my mother. I immediately followed up using the blood glucose meter and the measurement result was 219, a tiny measuring difference that I can live with quite well. I was able to repeat this test on different days, and also with other people. Whenever I did, it showed clearly that an inner state of calm was a decisive quality factor. Of course, a number of times I also failed in applying these tests.

Helmut H., farmer

Reducing the dose of my medication

In consultation and agreement with my doctor, I was able to reduce the dose of my medication (L-Thyroxin) by nearly half within a year, testing consistently every morning. I was prescribed and roughly adjusted to a daily dose of 125 mg, but it appeared that my need varied. Now my daily dose is between 60 and 75 mg and my blood values are fine.

Gisela G., retiree

Weight Loss

Before you try the fifth diet to lose weight, ask yourself whether it's really going to help you. Food satisfies our need for energy. But there are also other options: people who are newly in love can live on love alone.

There are four different stages of our energy level:

Stage 1: Your energy level is so low that in order to survive, food practically serves as your only source of energy while you keep gaining weight. Eating as doping to survive.

Stage 2: You have a higher energy level. Your weight doesn't change although you eat normal quantities. You don't manage to lose weight.

Stage 3: You have a high energy level, like people who are newly in love. You need little food and can lose weight easily.

Stage 4: You can live on light.

Test your energy level and find out how you can move up. Then, losing weight comes by itself.

Consider that allergic reactions to food account for about 40 per cent of overweight cases. This is primarily due to cow protein (milk, cheese, beef, etc), chicken protein (eggs, chicken meat) and wheat.

When the body experiences an allergic reaction, acid is produced and consequently water is retained to act as a buffer. If squeezing the skin firmly between your thumb and index finger at one of your forearms creates pain, the tissue is too sour and certainly retains extra water.

- Am I able to lose weight now?

- My energy level is at stage............

- Do I need my weight as a protection?

- Do I compensate for something with food?

- Is my excess weight primarily caused by retained water because I'm allergic to something?

- Should I omit this or that to lose weight?

Determining Allergens Using the Lie Detector

Who doesn't know the feeling of burning eyes when washing your hair? This is caused by highly allergenic preservatives called parabens; organic shampoos often contain them as well.

The only thing that helps here is looking at the list of ingredients and testing to err on the safe side. It's best to go through all the products in your bathroom and test them. Only those products that don't cause any stress should stay; the rest you should throw out. Or do you want to poison yourself and keep having red eyes after washing your hair, or put your beauty at stake?

Simply test everything:

- I tolerate this... (toothpaste, moist toilet paper, cream, shampoo, conditioner, soap)

Health and Beauty Products for All Users

For years, I have been developing or improving on products for pharmaceutical and cosmetics companies in different countries. Product development times can often be reduced to a fraction of the usual time by using the arm-length test and applying the related sensing abilities and perception. Without many trials and errors I can achieve an optimal result.

For example, this is how a toothpaste that consists of 35 essential oils was created, finely tuned to the acupuncture meridians that end at the teeth.

- Is this an optimal product for all users?

- Is this product harmful for any user?

- Are ingredients missing?

- Does it contain too many ingredients?

- Is this the right dose of ingredients?

Contaminated organic cosmetic cream

I had developed an organic cosmetic cream line and was just about to start large-scale production. That was when I met Uwe, and he quickly tuned in to the cream, sensed it and tested it. I only had to think about it, as I didn't have any of it with me. The testing revealed an allergic reaction. Doing in-depth testing, he was able to determine that the cream base contained the preservative paraben. I was really surprised, since the manufacturer had assured me that it didn't contain any preservatives.

The next day I called them, and heard that they had indeed added paraben, because 'that's how it's done.'

And so the cream base could still be altered just in time to avoid any allergic reactions by customers. This talent to test products and situations is really very impressive!

Jenny T., owner of a cosmetics company

Stress in Your Teeth

About 30 per cent of all people use toothpaste they don't tolerate. That's why it's good to test it. But it would also be good to test the dental materials used in your teeth.

Place your tongue on a filling and test it. Test several times in a row, because frequently, people are actually allergic to the materials used.

When your arms reveal stress caused by intolerance, or an allergic reaction, it's often only the beginning of the problem. Now you need to find a dentist who believes you and is able to help you. You would be surprised how many illnesses can be caused by dental materials. These include autoimmune diseases, intestinal or skin diseases, and asthma.

This is due to the fact that many people have an allergic reaction to amalgam, or they don't tolerate the palladium contained in less expensive dental gold. Methacrylates used in the plastics and glues also don't work for everyone. All substances used in dental materials whose content is below 1 per cent don't have to be declared. For this reason, the list of ingredients provided for dental material often doesn't help either, only testing does.

The best thing to do is test the dental materials at your dentist's before they enter your mouth. Ask the dentist to place on your throat any dental material he or she intends to use, and then test it. It's important that you also test the glues, sub-fillings and anaesthetics. Imagine having a particular dental material in your mouth and test it.

Doctors Can Be Convinced, Too

You need a bit of courage, or a medical doctor who is open to holistic medicine. Normally, you will be prescribed medication by your doctor to support you against a certain illness. You can take it and see which effects or side effects it has on you.

Or you can test it at the doctor's practice if your physician doesn't do it him- or herself.

- This medication or remedy helps me.

- I need this medication or remedy.

- I tolerate this medication or remedy.

Now you only need to have some backbone and assert your test results. But more and more physicians are open to new ideas in diagnostics and therapy.

A diagnostic method

In our diagnostic pyramid, the arm-length test offers the quickest form of diagnosis.

I can see the smallest changes often long before a laboratory test or X-ray machine can find them, and right away, I can test the optimal treatment, too.

In addition, I can use the arm-length test to test on all levels: physically, emotionally, mentally and energetically. This is unique in medicine.

Gabriele M., physician

At a practice for internal medicine

I'm a physician and learned to use the arm-length test over ten years ago.

At the time, I was looking for a usable kinesiological testing method that was easy to learn and would allow me to test individually and reliably medication, dosage and the duration of therapy.

Working with the arm-length test by far exceeded all my expectations.

Of course, practice makes perfect, but the arm-length test is a universal measuring tool. It's really easy to learn and it can be applied by practically *anybody in their daily life and at work, and naturally, also by me in my daily medical work.*

For us adults, trying out new things is usually a challenge. It's different for children. What's surprising to us is their lightness and speed when it comes to things they can easily understand.

There was a situation where I felt unable to make a decision. Then my daughter Marie-Kristin surprised me as she pointed out, 'Just ask your hands what's right!'

She has frequently seen that her arms differ in length when she is sick or stressed, and she feels a lot better when I can help her balance this.

The arm-length test has become an integral part of my medical practice and I can't imagine doing without it anymore.

Without words, it tells me a lot about the patient. And it's the best way to check the selected therapeutic options.

For me as a therapist, this test is intuition in its visible form and thus the sixth sense.

Time and again, I'm amazed by how easily and reliably it works.

Helge J., Specialist in internal medicine

Test using the arms

I worked with a patient who had been mountain climbing. On the mountain, he and his girlfriend were caught by surprise in a heavy storm and had to hold out on a ledge for the whole night.

She was able to squat, he had to stand up.

They descended the next morning.

A few weeks later, he came to see me in my practice. He wasn't doing well and had had trouble sleeping. He also had anxiety, which was usually not an issue for him. He's been alpine climbing for years.

The first test question was: 'I am I?'

Response: 'no'.

The second question was: 'I am dead?'

Response: 'yes'.

During that night, he had given up on himself.

After a full Innerwise treatment, he regained his clarity. The identity matched, he was back in life and was able to feel it, too.

A few days later, I received the following mail: 'Thank you, Oli, I'm fully back. When can you give a treatment to my girlfriend?'

Oliver D., Alternative health practitioner

THE ARM-LENGTH TEST FOR HAPPINESS AND WELLBEING

Good Luck and Positive Focus

'Happiness comes to the happy,' says Connor Mayfield. If you replace the negative focus which determines your life, and that of so many people, with a positive focus, the glass is no longer half-empty but half-full, and you will be happy.

Any meditation technique can support you in finding peace with yourself and your life.

- I'm happy.

- Life is beautiful.

- I'm grateful for all life experiences.

- I can see the lovable core in each human being.

- I'm responsible only for myself.

Am I Rich?

Wealth comes to those who feel wealthy. It comes to those who consider themselves rich in experience, abilities, skills and values. And to those who can accept their inner wealth, and have left behind their consciousness of what may be lacking.

And anybody can.

- I'm rich.

- I love to be successful.

- I'm worth being successful.

- Honesty and integrity are important to me.

- I love money.

Treating Yourself to Something Nice

It's time to treat yourself to something nice again. And it should be good for your health. But what? Which provider really delivers what he promises? What do you really need for your wellbeing? Frequently, it's going to be something different than you thought it would be.

Yoga or tai chi?

Facing the question 'yoga or tai chi workshop?' I didn't want to believe the test. Tai chi revealed stress, although it was my favourite choice!

So I still registered for the tai chi workshop. Two weeks later, I received an e-mail saying that the workshop wasn't going to take place.

Elisabeth G., speech therapist

Seeing Better, Looking Better

Which glasses suit me? What look am I going for? Professional, elegant, alternative or a little bit of everything?

Do you recognize that feeling? To me, choosing glasses is a real challenge. Your whole image is at stake.

Fortunately, there's the arm-length test in addition to the mirror.

Meike's glasses

'I can't see that well anymore. Mum, can you come to the optician's with me?'

When I looked into it using the arm-length test, it turned out that an additional 0.25 diopters for each eye would be better. The optician obtained the same results with his equipment. Out of a wide range of frames, and with the support of the arm-length test, we then selected the ideal ones. Today the glasses are ready and can be picked up.

A side effect: the optician took great interest in the testing and wanted to know more about it. Consequently, he asked me if I could test the place where he sleeps and also wait for his wife to return and test hers. Both were confirmed in their feeling: one in a positive and the other in a negative one.

Christiane L., coach

Christiane's glasses

For some time, I felt that my vision had improved. Using the arm-length test, I measured an improvement of 0.25 diopters in the one eye and of 0.5 in the other eye. The optician obtained the same results in his examination. A few days ago, I picked up my new glasses and can see perfectly.

Christiane L., coach

Following Spiritual Traditions

There is hardly any area in our new-age life, true wisdom apart, that is not also about manipulation, power, energy vampirism or hunting for souls.

It follows in the footsteps of the good old traditions of the ancient religions that have been practising this for so long.

Many techniques, such as reiki and shamanic practices, and also certain yoga styles, work with initiations and related variations. Therefore, it's crucial to test them in advance. In such rituals, people are connected to energies and beliefs that can alter their lives in a negative way and are often hard to get rid of.

- Is this offer based on integrity?

- Is the teacher at eye-to-eye level with me (where a good teacher should be)?

- Is the energy that I'm connected to clean, clear and honest?

- Is this really a fair price that I'm paying for this connection?

- Does this offer serve my growth?

- Does it respect my freedom?

- Will my inner light grow on this path?

- Will I become dependent?

- Will I be used?

- Is the offer honest and free of manipulation?

- Is there a better way for me?

- Do I need this experience for my growth?

- Is the person I get involved with authentic?

Yoga ashram

Once, I found myself in an existential crisis and wanted to take refuge in a yoga ashram in Germany; at the time, I didn't feel strong enough to take care of myself.

Some friends told me about a large ashram, and also about their admission ritual. It involved a test and swearing to a mantra. As I imagined taking part in this ritual, the arm-length test revealed a panic reaction. So, I decided to travel by myself to Italy for two months to paint. And when I returned home, I felt I had healed.

Later on, people who had taken part in the ashram's admission ritual told me that they all experienced a dramatic loss of life energy afterwards. They also reported that all of the ashram's staff and managers who had worked there for more than two years had fallen ill. Thus, the arm-length test helped me to regain my strength and power.

Sabine I., yoga teacher

THE ARM-LENGTH TEST IN RELATIONSHIPS

Love and Partnership

This topic is a large playground for arm-length test aficionados:

- Do I love myself?

- Do I love my partner?

- Have we got entangled in certain patterns?

- Are we honest with one another?

- Do I feel like having sex today?

- Can I unfold myself in this relationship?

- Am I dependent?

- Do I lose energy through this person?

- Do I live on the energy of others?

- Can I trust my partner 100 per cent?

Finding the Right Partner

With this test, finding a partner is really easy! Since attraction is based on resonance and a decision of the heart, the arm-length test is the best guide – much better than the pelvic area, the eyes or the mind. Unless you are just looking for somebody to spend the night with, to show off with or to argue with.

- Is this the right partner for me?

- Are we a good match?

- Are we meant to get together?

- Is it already the right time?

- Should I talk to him/her now?

The Relationship Check-up

As we fall in love, the great illusion of being one often doesn't last very long. What follows is a relationship that often turns into mutual dependencies.

Many relationships would long be over if both partners were honest with themselves and didn't cling on to the relationship for the sake of security. But everyone has to decide for him- or herself how many compromises they are willing to make. And usually, hope dies last.

The person I fell in love with and with whom I now share my life is:

- My love

- My husband/wife/child

- An object of manipulation and control

- My future ex-partner

- My friend

Reconnecting

I use the arm-length test as an anchor to reassure me. It reconnects me. Time and again, it confirms that I can trust my feelings and intuitions.

Tina A., educator

Dynamics Between Parents and Children

Who actually bears responsibility for the family?

That's pretty clear, you will say; the parents, of course. That's true. In the optimal case – that is, sometimes.

If a child bears the main responsibility, it's not surprising if he or she behaves like an overwhelmed adult. If only one of the adults bears the responsibility, the partner is often perceived as another child. It depends on the social maturity of all involved, which often leads to unpredictable behaviour.

In our family, the one who bears the largest responsibility is:

- Me

- My partner

- My child/children

Where is my partner at this moment?

One day, I had an idea – to find out where Kristina was located at that very moment by using the arm-length test. We were both in Vienna and had arranged to meet and take the same train home. We hadn't decided yet whether to hop on the train at the same stop. I connected myself to Kristina and asked where she was right then. The scope of potential locations was manageable. For each location, I used the arm-length test, asking if Kristina was there. If she wasn't there, I went on to the next location and tested again.

I was looking for Kristina at the train station 'Spittelau' but couldn't see her there.

– So I asked if she was there? No.

– At the railway station 'Franz-Josefs-Bahnhof'? Yes.

– In the last car? No.

– In the second-to-last car? Yes.

– At the lower level of the second-to-last car? No.

– At the upper level of the second-to-last car? Yes.

I called her on her mobile phone and told her what I'd tested. And it was exactly right.

Kristina then asked me if I also knew whether she was by herself or with somebody else. So I tested but couldn't find my inner calm anymore and started to doubt myself. One time it was a 'yes', then a very small 'no'… the picture was quite restless. Perhaps this was also related to the fact that Melanie had to get off the train at Heiligenstadt (one stop after Spittelau).

Herbert H., administrative official

The lie detector for kids

Immediately after taking the Innerwise basic workshop, I integrated the arm-length test into my daily life. What should I wear today, or which shampoo, cream, etc. can I tolerate?

The way I deal with my children (13 and 7 years old) has also changed. When they have an argument and both think they are right, of course we use the arm-length test. Since the children know that it works, more and more often they come around before the test is used. Even telling little fibs is no longer that easy for my kids; in most situations, it's enough when I say, 'Well, we can just test this.' And, we have a lot of fun each time!

And it also works the other round as a way for my children to put something across to me that my mind can't or doesn't want to believe. Then they say, 'Just test it with us!'

In July, the kids attended the Innerwise children's workshop. There, they learned how to use the arm-length test themselves. Since then, they have started to use it on their own here and there.

It's also a good way for me to see where I stand right now. Prior to each test, I always ask if I'm able to test; in this way, I realize very quickly when I'm out of balance. Thus, the test only confirms what my feeling is trying to communicate.

Claudia R., designer

An arm-length testing frenzy

We are in a real arm-length test frenzy at home. Frieda managed to find out exactly how expensive Mum's new shoes, jewellery, etc. were, and her friends at school are already using it, too. Jan was even able to talk my husband into applying the test, predicting that Dad wasn't going to be stuck in traffic today (and of course, he was right). And naturally I also test all sorts of possible and impossible things and the children respect the reliable lie detector. As you can see, we are having lots of fun!

Heike K., physician

Testing Your Social Maturity

If you suddenly behave like a 12-year-old when visiting your parents, at that moment your social maturity is 12 years. At work/in the office, it will probably match your real age, such as 43 years, for instance.

Social maturity indicates how we behave. It should more or less match our real age. If it differs by a few years, that's still OK though.

Also, it should remain about the same in all life situations.

A reality we often encounter in life is that a six-year-old child behaves like a 25-year-old because the parents act like five-year-olds, and someone in the family has to assume responsibility. Or a 37-year-old behaves like a 15-year-old and doesn't take responsibility for his life. But that's not healthy.

Social maturity is tested in years:

- When I'm by myself, my social maturity is:

- When I'm with my partner, my social maturity is:

- At work, my social maturity is:

- When I have sex, my social maturity is:

- When I visit my parents, my social maturity is:

Can you see some things more clearly now?

Honesty is the Best Policy

Often, we have to decide whether to tell the whole truth or wriggle free of a situation with a big or a little lie. It's just that, sooner or later, these lies return to haunt us.

Our very first responsibility is to be honest with ourselves; if we aren't, our lies make us sick.

It's not our responsibility whether the other person is able to cope with our honesty.

- Should I tell the whole truth now?

- Is this lie healthy for me?

- Is being honest also better for the other person?

THE ARM-LENGTH TEST AT HOME

Finding the Right Home

Finding a home where your entire family feels good, and where everybody is able to recharge their batteries – in short, finding the best environment for your family life – is often a decision you take for years to come. During testing, it's important to think not only of the current moment but of the entire time that you intend to spend there, as well as all the people and animals who will be living there with you. What good does the best home do you if you want to live there with your partner but he or she can't stand it?

- Do I live in the right place?

- Should I move to a different place?

- Should I move out?

- Should I rent an apartment/a house?

- Should I buy an apartment/a house?

How long will it be until it starts raining?

One afternoon I wanted to go for a little walk, but it was pretty overcast. As I looked at the cloud formations, I wasn't quite sure whether these were rain clouds or whether they would simply drift away. So I thought to myself, why not connect to the clouds and ask them in how many minutes it would start raining here. I got the number eight.

I followed up by testing the minutes with the arm-length test and also got eight. Then I asked the clouds if we could still go for an eight-minute walk and return home dry. The response of the arm-length test was 'yes'.

Testing both nine and ten minutes, the response was already 'no', so we didn't go too far and returned home dry just before the eight minutes had passed. As we were entering the house, it started to drizzle; the eight minutes were over.

Julia L., student

Setting Up Your Home

Put the wardrobe here? And the bed there? Should this be the children's room? Rearranging the furniture? A new paint? Buying new furniture? Looking for a new home? Moving to a different country?

Imagine the purpose of the room – i.e. bedroom, dining room, office, creative space – and test if this room fulfills its purpose in an optimal way. If not, imagine changing something and test again.

Finding a Competent Tradesman

You only want to work with people who master their trade, love their work and offer good quality? Then go test it!

Testing craftsmen

I had big problems with various craftsmen and I didn't know how to fix the mess I was in. With Christiane, I tested what a solution would look like. The testing revealed that Mr Müller was key to this scenario, the number one so to speak. I called him and felt very relieved when he told me that he'd take care of my situation.

He managed to have everything organized within an hour, so that I had nothing else to do. Then he said, 'If anything else comes up, just call me first.' I really felt like telling him, 'Yes, I know. That's what we've tested.'

By 5 p.m. the craftsmen were at my door. Bingo!

Everything went so smoothly, almost by itself! Two weeks later the next craftsman, who I'd been waiting for in vain for several weeks, showed up. This time, I insisted that the master himself would take care of the repair (another result of the testing). Before, two of his workers had worked for six hours without fixing the damage satisfactorily. It was all taken care of in an hour this time around. It was great! All my frustration, my distress and worries were gone.

Maik W., broker

THE ARM-LENGTH TEST AT WORK AND FOR STUDY

Creative Thinking

My favourite pastime is thinking. It constantly produces the craziest ideas, so I test them to find out which are worth pursuing.

First comes the thought, then my arms check its usefulness and potential success. A positive response gets it into the second round for deeper reflection.

Living yourself

Since I started to use the arm-length test, my work has been changing more and more toward 'I'm becoming myself, that is, who I am.' Fortunately!!!

Christiane L., coach

Efficiency at Home and at Work

Work should be effective and efficient *and* fun! The only thing that can help here is good planning. And who would know best what to do when? Yes, that's right: the omniscient subconscious!

Ask your subconscious, and take care of your tasks in the order you tested. You will feel that things go much more smoothly.

- Should I water the plants today?

- Should I reply to this letter today?

- Should I make this call today?

- Should I read my e-mails first?

- Do I really have to take care of this today?

- Is my girlfriend ready to talk? Should I call her now?

- Which book should I read today?

Is this person available to talk to me right now?

I'm often in a situation where I need to know if a specific person has time to discuss something, or

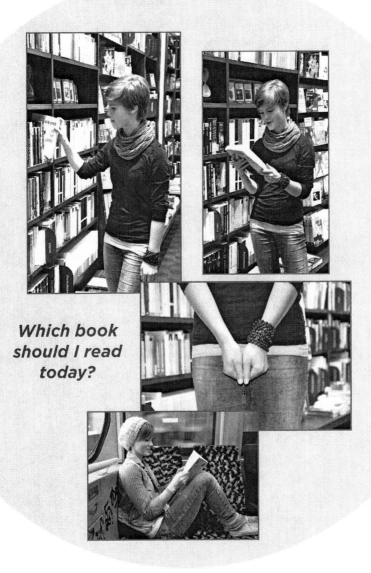

Which book should I read today?

talk to me on the phone right then. Of course, one could call and ask if the person is available to talk. But I thought to myself, 'Why not ask that person first in my mind if he or she is available, and then test using the arm-length test?' At the beginning, I also called them up afterwards to verify if the response I had received from the arm-length test was correct. It's amazing and wonderful to discover that these answers are always right. In many instances, this saves me listening to their phone's mailbox or going over to see them.

Robert E., manager

In the Team Flow

In team meetings, everyone tests upcoming decisions with his or her arms. Then, results are compared and decisions made. Whenever this procedure has been applied, it has led to optimal project results and saved a great deal of time.

Finding my own answers

Since I got to know the arm-length test through different therapists who worked with me, I kept asking myself if I couldn't also test myself using this test.

Sporadically, I asked myself easy little questions. Just for fun, I imagined how I'd pass on this question to my subconscious.

Therefore, I was all the more surprised about the answers. With time, they clearly empowered me and boosted my courage in handling situations in my daily life, at work and in dealing with other people.

I was slowly gaining more and more confidence in myself as well as my responses.

I very often encounter situations in my job where I'm not sure how to react: better this way or that way? Better 'left' or 'right'?! Then, I often think I don't know the right answer. I have learned, however, to ask myself using the arm-length test. And I've also learned to trust its – my very own – responses. With time, I realized that the answer lies within me.

Small things in my daily life or tricky situations at work – no matter which life situation is giving me a hard time at a given moment – I know there is always somebody at my side who I can ask and whose answers I can trust! It's not simply a gut feeling that I'm referring to. It's a confirmation that I'm on the right path.

Stefanie E., business consultant

Living Your Calling

We should not simply practise a profession or do a job, but instead live our calling. Doing this makes us happy, it fulfils us, and we can enjoy what we do for a living.

When choosing your profession, imagine yourself practising it and then test. It could also be that you obtain a 'yes' only on the related education or training. In that case, it's meant to be a valuable experience for you.

- My profession is my calling.

- Work is a necessary evil.

- Is it a compromise that provides security but doesn't fulfil me, nor challenge or satisfy me?

- I love my work.

- I'm good at it.

- I enjoy taking responsibility for tasks.

- My work is a burden.

- My work challenges me and allows me to grow.

- I accomplish my tasks with a high degree of quality.

146

Using the arm-length test to find your calling

My wife recommended me to attend an Innerwise basic workshop, where I learned the arm-length test. It was a totally new world for me.

Immediately after the course, I started to test everything: toothpaste, shower gel, shaving cream, skin care, shampoo, etc.

Testing different food was also very interesting. I tested bread. It was OK. White bread rolls: OK. Soy products: stress. Baking agents: stress. That's interesting, I thought.

And then I thought of testing people. I thought of my parents: OK. My mother-in-law: OK... whew, I was lucky! I remembered my time in school, and all of a sudden I experienced a high level of stress. I carried on testing when I went shopping at the supermarket.

Now once more back to the Innerwise workshop that completely changed my life and the way I perceive and look at the world. To me, it was so fascinating that I decided to continue with the training, and there I found my calling.

Today, I'm self-employed and work as an Innerwise practitioner and mentor in Austria. I'm grateful to

Uwe Albrecht for this wonderful system that has enabled me to live my calling.

Robert P., mentor

Studying Can Be So Simple

There are several reasons why studying can be difficult. There is an inner resistance against the subject or the teacher; you are sitting in a bad place with, for example, geopathic stress that makes you feel you have to move the whole time; there is bad lighting in the room; or you are sitting next to the wrong people. Sometimes, the rooms at school are also designed or set up in such a way that it's difficult to concentrate. Only the most resilient students can keep sufficient focus to follow the lesson. Another important cause when somebody has trouble studying can be insufficient sleep due to electrosmog (AC electric fields), resulting in chronic fatigue.

Or they may be wearing the wrong colour and feeling uncomfortable as a result. Or they may be at the wrong school...

- I want to learn.

- I'm sitting in a place that is good for me.

- Would it be good for me to take a break?

- I get along with my teachers.

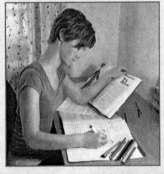

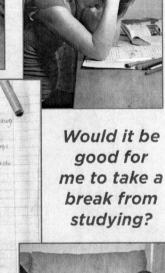

Would it be good for me to take a break from studying?

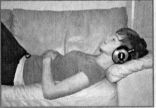

- My teachers have confidence in my ability to perform well.

- I select the following electives: ....

- I drop the following electives: ....

- Would it be good for me to change school?

Choosing the right seminar

Last Sunday, Meike had to register for her new lectures and seminars. She was spoilt for choice, but using the arm-length test, it was possible to select the courses that fitted her best within minutes. Although some didn't seem to make sense at first, when looking at the whole picture they did and they felt right. This set the mood for the new semester!

Christa F., psychologist

THE ARM-LENGTH TEST FOR ANIMALS AND PETS

Communicating with Animals

As we cannot talk to animals directly, except for some animal whisperers, you can often test dogs and cats directly using their paws. Testing also works if you test on behalf of the animal using your own arms. Tune in to the animal, apply spherical vision and ask:

- Is my animal happy?

- Is my animal healthy?

- Does my animal need anything?

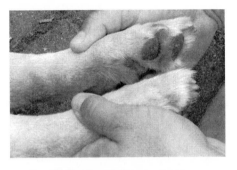

Polly the dog says 'yes'

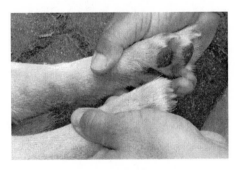

Polly the dog says 'no'

Communicating with our cat

Three years ago, we got a lovely cat. Sometimes it's difficult to understand what our cat wants from us. With the arm-length test, it has become a lot easier to communicate with her. When our cat meows, we test a few questions. This way, we know more precisely what she wants.

Ulrike K., marketing director

Treating Animals

This is a lot of fun, because animals react immediately and with gratitude. Imagine you are your animal and think of its hips, if it has hip problems. Your arms differ in length. Then think of a remedy, or of changing its food, or of more or different physical activities, or of minerals and vitamins. The stress will disappear with the right answer. Now you know that you are on the right track.

If your animal needs to be vaccinated, you can also ask when you should do it and whether a certain date is really the best one for your animal.

In this way, you can test your animal's physical and emotional state and frequently find remedies yourself.

Please bear in mind that with animals, the cause of a problem can often be found in their owner; out of love, animals take over an emotional burden or even physical illness. For that reason, start first with yourself and don't forget to apply spherical vision so that you don't deceive yourself.

- Is the animal's problem related to the people it belongs to? Do the people need help first?

Miraculous healing of a horse

Our horse, a mare, had a leg injury and hadn't eaten anything for days.

I took the Innerwise healing cards and let her smell them. In this way, she already took what she needed.

Then I tested her using my own arms and added a few frequencies (Innerwise healing cards), which I put on her belly. She stopped foundering and started to eat again. And everybody was amazed.

Kerstin H., energy practitioner

THE ARM-LENGTH TEST IN EVERYDAY SITUATIONS

Choosing a Holiday Destination

Don't you agree that the whole concept of going on holiday is pretty questionable?

That is, doing a job for eleven months that you don't really enjoy and then taking one month to recover from it? To me, there's something sick about that.

Rather than allowing us to recover from our work, holidays should offer an opportunity to find inspiration and creativity, discover new things and allow the unexpected to happen.

If you have fun working, it also gives you energy, it doesn't just take energy. Then you no longer need to go on holiday in order to recharge your batteries.

The world is so rich and has so much to offer! There are plenty of different ways to live, think, be... and we have the unique chance to be able to experience all this by travelling and engaging in something new.

Off you go, get rich!

- It's time for a holiday! But where to? Should I go to an island?

- Where is life's next adventure awaiting me?

- What kind of holiday is best for me?

- Should I book the flight only and look for accommodation on site?

- Should I travel alone or with somebody?

Checking in at the airport

There was a huge queue at all the check-in counters in Leipzig airport. Of all counters, we were standing in line at the one moving the slowest, because a trainee was receiving his first hands-on training. My husband was getting impatient and wanted to change lines. But I tested it with my arms and told him, 'Let's stay here. It's good for us, although I don't know why yet.'

And it paid off. We got seats with more legroom. On other airlines, that usually costs extra. The trainer pointed this out to the trainee, and my husband, who is tall, was really glad about that! On our flight back, we were once more able to benefit from this information.

Karen J., musician

Looking for a store in a foreign city

Last year, we went to Iceland and visited the capital, Reykjavik. A friend had asked us to bring back for her 'Swiss Miss with Marshmallows', which you can't find in Germany. We had little time and didn't know Reykjavik, and we didn't have a map of the city either.

Using the arm-length test, we tested if there was a store where they'd sell 'Swiss Miss' within a 15-minute walk of where we were. Then we tested the direction we should take.

After a few changes in direction, we passed a small supermarket which sold 'Swiss Miss' but without marshmallows. Well, we had been a bit imprecise in how we phrased the question...

So we asked about 'Swiss Miss with Marshmallows' and went off to a bigger supermarket where we found the product our friend had asked for.

Marion O., actress

Carpooling: looking for a ride

In September, I decided for the first time to look for carpooling offers. I was looking for a ride from Dresden to Karlsruhe and back and was in the position to choose between two drivers. Based on the arm-length test result, I decided to go for the option which was much less convenient time-wise, but in hindsight, turned out to be the jackpot. It was a driver from Dresden who, at 1.30 a.m., dropped me off right at my door.

Monika F., retiree

Premonition at the airport

When we arrived at the airport in Leipzig, we were picked up by a shuttle bus that was supposed to drop us off at the car park. The driver asked if it was OK for us to wait a little longer so that he could pick up a passenger who was arriving with the flight from Frankfurt. At first, I was fine, but after a while, I decided to check with the arm-length test if the other passenger was still coming. The answer was 'no'. When I asked the driver if we could leave, he didn't respond. About 20 minutes later, he finally contacted airport information and found out that, because of missing luggage, the passenger was still busy at the baggage claim.

Birgit O., nurse

Before Casting Your Vote...

Before filling out your ballot paper and casting your vote...

Hold on a moment and savour these words...

You cast your vote, which is your voice, and simply deposit it in a ballot box. Does this match your understanding of democracy? So... before you go ahead and do this, you should test who you really want as your representative. Somebody who feigns and lies and is only interested in his or her power? Or do you vote for somebody who represents your interests in an honest manner; somebody who shows character and integrity and doesn't stab you in the back later on?

Simply test it. Look at the promises on the election posters and ask yourself whether they will be kept. Listen to the candidates' election speeches and simply test whether it's the truth or a lie.

The Election Check:

- Can I trust this person?

- Will this person keep his/her promises?

- Are my interests important to that person?

- Will I be used for personal power interests?

- Does this office only serve to offer financial security to this person and give his life a purpose?

- Is this person honest?

- Should I vote for this person/party?

- Is there somebody better?

- If there is no better candidate, is this candidate/ party the smallest compromise that I'm willing to make?

A strange experience with the arm-length test

I had a strange experience using the arm-length test with my friend Klaus, who is a very sensitive person. He had asked me to test a few questions that were critical to his life path. After going through a few questions we felt that the arm-length test was being manipulated. Klaus told me immediately that something wasn't right with the test. It was as if somebody was pulling his arm muscle as the question was asked. When the question was asked again, what felt like manipulation before was not present anymore.

It was only a bit later that it dawned on me – this feeling of manipulation had occurred when asking questions about the future, or when we had entered a dead end with our question. The arm-length test confirmed this at a later stage.

If we had applied spherical vision during testing, we would always have received clear answers. We had also forgotten to test if we were even allowed to ask these questions about the future.

Peter M., politician

Crime Detection

It's only a matter of time before the arm-length test is used as a lie detector by the police and in court.

Turning detective in the hotel room

My parents and I were staying overnight in a hotel. At first glance, my parents' room was friendlier, brighter and smelled better. My room, a single room, was musty and seemed darker. It just wasn't that nice. But it was clean, so on the whole OK.

There was a fan heater above the bathroom door where I detected traces of smeared blood and tiny blood splatters. Out of curiosity, I used the arm-length test. These were the responses I got when I checked out the following questions:

– Did a murder take place in this hotel room? No.

– Did somebody get physically harmed in this hotel room? Yes.

– Did anybody die in this bathroom? Yes.

– Were the regular police in this bathroom? No.

– Were the criminal police in this bathroom? Yes.

– Did a woman kill her husband? No.

– Did a man kill his wife? No.

– Did a man kill another man? Yes.

– Was the killing motivated by relationship issues? No.

– Was it about business issues? Yes.

– Did it happen at night? Yes.

– Was it about money? No.

– I checked different motives...

– Was it about cars? Yes.

– I checked different countries: the offender was Polish.

– Again, I went through different countries: the victim was German.

– *Age: both young men.*

– *Time of the crime (I looked at years and seasons): September 2009.*

– *Did the victim accompany the offender into his hotel room? Yes.*

– *Is the offender known, but not caught yet? Yes.*

– *Weapon used in the crime (I checked out the material, length, whether it was a weapon, a tool or a kitchen utensil): metal, 6 cm (2.4 in), pointed tip at both ends, what exactly... I stopped testing.*

– *Does the offender currently live in a German city? Yes.*

– *I went through the letters: J.E.D... I stopped testing since my concentration was gone.*

– *Does the hotel reception know about it? Yes.*

I don't know if it's possible to test such things with the arm-length test. The results were clear, without ambiguity, and I also cross-checked every time. When I checked the internet, I couldn't find any indication of a murder that would have occurred in this hotel in September 2009. What I do know is that there was blood on the fan heater above the bathroom door.

Uta K., industrial business management assistant

Who Lies the Most?

This is a fun pastime for the whole family. Every night, just in time for the news, everyone goes in testing position. Then we test the degree of truth of the news of the day.

- Is this news true?

- Is there a lie in this piece of news?

- Is this piece of news aimed at manipulating people?

Internalizing the arm-length test

In the beginning, I tested everything: food, people, rooms, objects – simply everything. As a result, I now hardly need the test anymore, because I increasingly trust my intuition and can follow my first impulse without letting limiting thoughts take over.

Also, when working with clients, I need the arm-length test less and less. I feel what's coming; I 'see' it. It's as if I'm applying the test internally without having to consult the other person. And when I check using the test, it fits.

Theresa G., therapist

This is a small selection of the options this wonderful tool offers us.

The arm-length test has changed my life and has made me a happier, healthier and more creative person.

Have fun exploring and discovering all about it!

Chapter 5

THE ARM-LENGTH TEST: AN OVERVIEW

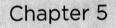

SPHERICAL VISION

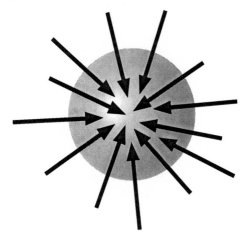

Look at the topic from all directions, just like the arrows that are pointing to the centre from all directions in the illustration above.

THE ARM-LENGTH TEST

1. Regular test

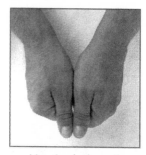

Yes (or balance)

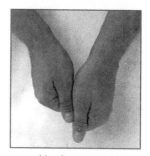

No (or stress)

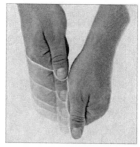

Allergy or panic response

2. Initial stress: treat yourself

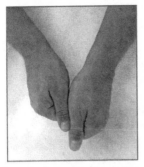

*Arm-length test shows 'no', or stress response,
with 'yes' statement*

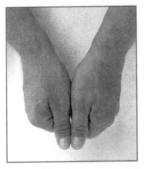

*Arm-length test shows what seems to be a 'yes',
or balance, with 'no' statement*

3. Blockage/rigidity: treat yourself

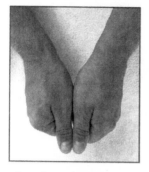

*Arm-length test: 'yes',
or balance*

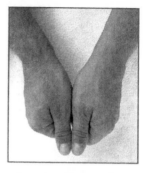

*Arm-length test: 'no',
or stress*

Or

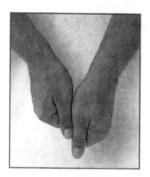

*Arm-length test shows 'no',
or stress response,
with 'yes' statement*

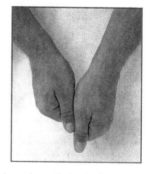

*Arm-length test shows 'no',
or stress response,
with 'no' statement*

STRESS/RIGIDITY/BLOCKAGE: TREATING YOURSELF

When you think of the right remedy and imagine applying it, the stress disappears and the rigidity is dissolved.

Remedies and ways to support healing:

- Drinking water
- Changing the colour of your clothes
- Imagining beautiful situations or colours
- Listening to music
- Speaking the truth
- Meditating
- Practising yoga
- Painting
- Taking a shower
- Smelling flowers
- Drinking herbal tea
- Dancing
- Meditating with crystals
- Using Bach flower essences or homeopathy
- Going for a walk

or

- Treating yourself with *Innerwise®: The Complete Healing System*

TESTING

Always do the pre-tests:

- Say 'yes' and test – your (and the test subject's) arms should be equally long.

- Say 'no' and test – your (and the test subject's) arms should differ in length.

- Always use spherical vision during testing.

- Am I allowed to test this? – yes/no.

- Will I receive a meaningful response? – yes/no.

Option 1: for Beginners

Make a statement or imagine something, then test.

- Your arms are equally long: no stress.

- The length of your arms differs: stress.

Option 2: for Advanced Practitioners

You can now test using both statements and questions. Here, assessing the response depends entirely on how the question is phrased.

Examples:

1. Should I do...?
2. Does... harm me?

If it really harms you, your arms are equally long. Your body says 'yes'.

*   Your arms are equally long: yes.
*   The length of your arms differs: no.

USING THE ARM-LENGTH TEST THROUGHOUT THE DAY

*   Should I get up now?
*   What should I wear today?
*   What's best for me to have for breakfast today?
*   How should I organize my work day in the most efficient way?
*   What's important to do today?

- What should I do first?

- What should I eat today?

- What should I buy?

- What should I do with the kids today?

- What do I need to feel good today?

- Should I really say this now?

- Which movie do I want to watch?

- Which book should I read today?

- Is my business partner reachable now?

- What should I prepare for tomorrow?

CONTACT AND FURTHER INFORMATION

Videos on the Arm-Length Test

You can find videos on the arm-length test on my website, www.innerwise.eu, or on www.youtube.com.

Workshops on the Arm-Length Test and on Innerwise

The *Innerwise* Institute offers workshops in several countries.

For further information and dates of workshops, please visit www.innerwise.eu or contact us at info@innerwise.eu

By the Same Author

Innerwise®: The Complete Healing System (Hay House, 2012)

NOTES

ABOUT THE AUTHOR

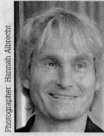

Uwe Albrecht was born in East Germany in 1966. He is a physician and pioneer of energy medicine. In addition to conventional medicine, Uwe studied traditional Chinese medicine (TCM), classical European healing methods, physioenergetics, osteopathic repositioning techniques (AORT), homeopathy, holistic biological medicine, emotional therapies and sacred geometry. Based on his findings, experiences and insights, Uwe developed Innerwise® as a healing system for all of life.

www.innerwise.eu

CPSIA information can be obtained at www.ICGtesting.com
Printed in the USA
LVOW13s0948071013

355737LV00001B/1/P